I0491673

B CELL IMMUNOTHERAPY IN ORAL CANCER
A SHORT REVIEW

Smitha T
Anela Thomas

ELIVA PRESS

ELIVA PRESS

Smitha T

Anela Thomas

As the emerging trend in therapeutics of cancer refocus on immunotherapy, it is one of the most effective measure to reduce the current rate of mortality and morbidity rate. Immunotherapy has been still at a progressive note for complete recovery of tumor and its recurrence. T cell based immunotherapy has been recognised for its role in curbing the tumor progression rate. Although, the role of B cells is still at controversy. Exploring both the antitumorogenic and protumorogenic responses in a tumor microenvironment emphasis this fact to reconsider the role of B lymphocyte.

Published: Eliva Press SRL
Address: MD-2060, bd.Cuza-Voda, 1/4, of. 21 Chişinău, Republica
Moldova
Email: info@elivapress.com
Website: www.elivapress.com

ISBN: 978-1-952751-43-1

TABLE OF CONTENTS

INTRODUCTION

Oral Squamous Cell Carcinoma (OSCC) is one among the commonest cancer occurring globally. The prevalence and incidence of OSCC is very frequently reported in various parts of Indian subcontinent[1]. Emerging treatment strategies are focused in finding a better cure for the disease so as to reduce its present load of mortality and morbidity.

Immunotherapy is one of the most important arenas in treating patients for better prognosis and reduced reoccurrence rate. The concept of immunotherapy is based on the body innate ability of *'immunosurveiliance'*. Immunosurveillance is defined as ability of body to recognise self and non-self. This is brought through the co-ordinated activities of both innate and acquired immunity. The principal cells that take part in this response are primarily B cells and T cells [2].

The immune response of both B cells and T cells is an indispensable entity present within the tumor microenvironment. The role of T-cells are been widely studied and discussed globally [3].CD8+ T cells utilize T cell receptors (TCRs) to recognize MHC-presented peptides and subsequently mount an antigen-specific cytolytic attack [4,5]. The Antigen–TCR engagement ultimately leads to the activation and proliferation of CD8+ T cells that play a crucial role in autoimmunity, response to pathogens, and tumor suppression [6,7]. Genetic rearrangement of TCRs during T cell development enables the recognition of a broad spectrum of processed Antigens in the adult immune system.

Antigens (Ags), typically foreign substances of environmental, viral, or bacterial origin, products of somatically altered proteins, or debris from dying (apoptotic) cells, are processed and presented by major histocompatibility complex (MHC) on Ag-presenting cells (APCs), including (but not limited to) dendritic cells, macrophages, and B cells [8]. Therefore, it is important to recognise the various types of cells associated with tumor microenvironment and their role in the progression of tumor spread.

The role of B lymphocytes is to discussed to implement them at the level of therapeutics. The various roles played by the B lymphocytes in tumor microenvironment are to be critically analysed and

2

evaluated. The controversial behaviour of B lymphocytes as pro-tumorogenic and anti-tumorogenic has not been validated still. At this instance discussing about subtypes and regulator cells and various B cell markers can be helpful in concluding the characteristic role played by B lymphocytes in tumor microenvironment.

The conclusiveness of the role played by the B lymphocytes in the tumor microenvironment has been too ruled out well to designate its potential in present scenario of therapeutics. However both pro-tumorogenic and anti-tumorogenic role played by the B lymphocytes can be instrumented in modulating the immunogenic response towards the tumor progression [9].

The pro-tumorigenic effects can be further enhanced to resist tumor invasion and reoccurrences of the tumor. Further, the anti-tumorigenic response when suppressed at its molecular level can ensure better treatment prognosis and survival rate in patients. Identifying the pathways modulating the immune response and recognising their regulatory elements is also considered an important entity is learning the tumor immune response of the body.

Immune escape mechanism of tumor and pattern switching character of the tumor becoming immune-resistant to common therapeutics are to be evaluated even critically at this point to find a cure. Immunotherapy to be implemented at the basic level should also establish its potentiality by evoking body's natural immune response and sustaining it through a long time preventing its relapses and reoccurrences.

Incrementing and implementing immunotherapeutic in conventional therapeutically measures can be the future of both diagnosis and therapeutics. In this context, discussing more on B lymphocytes and utilising it as therapeutic tool can also be considered promising.

ONTOGENY OF B LYMPHOCYTES

<u>B lymphocyte origin and differentiation</u>

The first stages of B Cell development take place in complex microenvironments created by the stromal cells of the bone marrow known as "niches" from which come the stimuli and factors

3

required to initiate a series of cell signals. IL-7 is critical to the development of the B Cells and is produced by the cells of the stroma. Various other molecules activate transcription factors that induce, or repress, the expression of different target genes that modulate cell survival, proliferation, and differentiation [10].

The development of the B Cells initiates from a haematopoietic stem cell (HSC). This transforms into an early lymphoid progenitor (ELP) and, then, becomes a common lymphoid progenitor (CLP) from which natural killer cells (NK) and dendritic cells (DC) [11] . The common lymphoid progenitor-2 (CLP-2), which is responsible for the B cell lineage. This is considered the first stage of the immature B cells [12].

A pre-requisite for the development of the B Cells in bone marrow is the absence or suppression of protein Notch-1 (N1) signalling, which is necessary for T Cell development . During the differentiation of the B Cells, a process of gene recombination is structured initially that codes for segments V (Variable), D (Diversity), and J (Joining) of the heavy chain (chain H) together with that of the genes for segments V and J of the light chain (chain L) of the membrane-bound immunoglobulin [13].

This recombination process is initiated by the complex of proteins RAG1- RAG2 that generate the rupture of the double chain of DNA between segments of genes and specific recognition sites that are also known as "recombination signal sequences." This process leads to the generation of B Cells that express a wide range of membrane bound immunoglobin. This will form the B Cell receptor (BCR) which is able to recognize more than 5 x 1013 different types of antigens [14].

During its development, the B Cell generates a wide diversity of BCR for the gene recombination process. Each cell has many allelic loci for the different BCR chains (two loci for the heavy chain and multiple loci for the light chain), each mature cell eventually expresses only a single type of receptor [14]. This is achieved by restricting the gene expression of the BCR of a single allele in a process known as allelic exclusion, which involves a mono-allelic activation and feedback inhibition.

4

The expression of pre-BCR is an important control point for the recombination of the heavy chain. Its product Igµ associates with a surrogate light chain (SLC), a heterodimer composed of two germline-encoded invariant proteins (V preB and λ5) to thus produce the molecular complex known as pre-BCR in the B Cell precursors [12,14]. Once this pre-BCR is expressed on the cell surface, it generates a signal that induces proliferation of the pre-B results in significant increase of number and carries out the heavy chain recombination. Furthermore, signalling through the pre-BCR is implicated in activation of the gene recombination for the light chain.

Based on the differential expression of a complex of surface markers, five stages (A, B, C, D and E) have been described for the development of immature B Cells that occur inside bone marrow. The stages are as follows: CLP-2 corresponds to stage A with expression of B220+, KIT-, CD19-, FLT3+, CD24low/-; CD43+, Ig M corresponds to early Pro-B cell with expression of B220+, KIT+, CD10+, CD19+, CD24+, CD43+, FLT3-, Ig M- stage C to late Pro-B cell which expresses BP1+. During stage D, the immature B Cell expresses a pre-receptor B (Igµ +SLC λ5 and V preB) which converts the cell into Pre-B with expression of B220+, CD19+, CD24+, CD25+, and CD43; and finally, stage E corresponds to the B immature cells with expression of B220+, CD19+, CD24+, CD43-, and Ig M+, which emerge from bone marrow and are guided towards the secondary lymphoid organs (spleen, lymph nodules, Payer's patches, tonsils, and mucosal tissue) to continue their differentiation into transitional B Cells (type 1 and type 2). The effect of molecules such as BAFF and APRIL, differentiate into marginal zone B Cells (MZB) or enter the germinal centers and microenvironment of cytokines that surrounds them, each of these cells transforms into a plasma Ab-secretory cell or memory B Cells transform into follicular B Cells (FoB). Later, depending on the Ag stimuli they receive the microenvironment of cytokines that surrounds them, each of these cells transforms into a plasma Ab-secretory cell or memory B Cells [15].

GERMINAL CENTRE FORMATION; B LYMPHOCYTE

Homing of B Cells in the spleen is regulated by expression of chemokines such as CCL21, CCL19, and CXCL13 produced by follicular dendritic cells (FDCs). These facilitate the movement of B Cells to the marginal zone or the follicles thereby giving rise to the formation of the germinal centers (GC). A GC is considered to be a specialized microenvironment of lymphoid tissue where an intense cell proliferation, somatic hypermutation, and selection by antigenic affinity occur. The early development of B Cell differentiation is completed and cells undergo apoptosis [16].

During this process, Tfh cells activate the B Cells, which proliferate and create the first part of a germinal center within the follicle. At this stage, somatic hyper mutation occurs (this is dependent on proliferation and the microenvironment of the germinal center although the exact factors that induce it are unknown). This process generates a progeny of B Cells with distinct receptors (almost identical but mutated in the variable zones). Some of these receptors do not recognize the presented Ag while others do with greater avidity. Where this maturation is happening, there are Ag-presenting DCs, and those B Cells that have increased their affinity for the Ag recognize it avidly and remain bound. This interaction is known as "maturation by affinity."

While the former happens, there is a change of BCR isotype through a process known as class-switch recombination (CSR), for which an intrachromosomal deletional rearrangement produces a change from the Cμ chain (which codes the constant region of IgM) to Cγ, Cα or Cε, encoding the constant regions of IgG, IgA, and IgE respectively [17]. Finally, different B Cells are generated with a BCR that has a specific isotype and a modified affinity for and exit to peripheral circulation. Some of these cells convert into plasma cells and go to the bone marrow (increasing the Igs) while others remain within the same lymphoid organ. Many other B Cells become memory B Cells. The germinal center forms at least one week after contact with the Ag [16].

B CELL RECEPTORS

The BCR is a macromolecular complex that is built in the membrane by IgM/ IgD with two additional Ig accessories denominated Ig α (CD79a) and Ig β (CD79b). The membrane-bound immunoglobulins are glycoproteins with a basic monomer. Each of these is made up of four polypeptide chains of which two are heavy (H) chains with a molecular weight of approx, 65 kDa, and the others are light (L) chains with a molecular weight of 25 kDa. Each L chain is linked to an H chain by a disulphuric bridge. The H chains are linked to each other by at least one other disulphuric bridge.

The IgM or IgD monomers correspond to the extracellular segments of the BCR. The two segments, the trans membranal and the intra-cytoplasmic, which result from an extension of the carboxy-terminal portion of the two H chains. The two V domains, which form the active sites allowing each BCR to bind specifically to an antigenic determinant, are found in the amino-terminal (H and L) portions of each peptide chain of the BCR. The antigen-BCR interaction is a non-covalent reaction [18]. The intra-cytoplasmic region of Ig, which presents only 3 amino acids (lysine-valine-lysine), is very small and does not permit to carry out the signaling process. The transmembranal segment of the C-terminal portion of the H chain of Ig consists of 25 amino acids found close to the protein tyrosine kinase (PTK) enzymes which, in turn, are close to the heterodimers.

SIGNALLING MECHANISMS

Stimulation of the B Cells via antigenic BCR begins with the recognition and capture of the Ag through BCR molecules. This induces their aggregation and triggers the signalling process by activating the SRC family kinase (SFK) which then phosphorylates the ITAM moieties of the accessory chains Igα and Igβ. They carry out the same function as the ζ chain (CD247) to activate the TCR and produce lipid-raft-associated calcium-signalling module forms .

This complex contains 3 classes of activated protein tyrosine kinases (PTKs):

i)   Lyn, Fyn, and Blk of the Src family;

ii)   Syk/ ZAP70;

iii)   of Bruton (Btk) of the Tec family

This initiates the formation of a macromolecular complex known as 'signalosome' composed of the BCR, the tyrosine kinases with some adaptor proteins such as CD19 and BLNK (B Cell linker protein), signalling enzymes such as the phospholipase C gamma - 2 (PLCγ2), the phosphatidylinositol 3-kinase (PI3K), and molecules of the Vav family. The signalling produced by the signalosome activates multiple signalling cascades which implicate other kinases, GTPases, and transcription factors such as NF-kB, Bcl6, NF-AT, FoxO, Jun, and ATF-2, etc [19]The activation of all these mechanisms gives rise to changes in cell metabolism, gene expression, and the organization of the cell cytoskeleton.

The state of maturation of the B Cells, the nature of the Ag, the magnitude and duration of signalling through the BCR, and the signals of other receptors such as CD40, the receptor of IL-21, and BAFF-R. Thus, many other trans membranal proteins such as CD45, CD19, CD22, PIR-B, and FcγRIIB1 (CD32) modulate specific elements of the signalling BCR.

During the in vivo processes, the B Cells are also activated by APCs, which capture and present the antigenic fractions on their cell surfaces. This type of B Cell activation by such cell membrane–associated Ags also requires a reorganization of the B Cell cytoskeleton. Thus, it is to be expected that the complexity of the signalling mediated by the BCR allows diverse biological effects to occur, including cell survival, tolerance, or apoptosis as well as proliferation and differentiation in Ab-producing cells or memory B Cells [20,21].

CO-RECEPTORS OF THE BCR

During B Cell activation, another series of molecules participates to build a molecular complex that acts as a BCR co-receptor. These molecules can significantly increase the signalling Induced initially by the BCR and include: CR2 (CD21), CD19, CD45, CD38, and CD81 [22,23]. The binding of CD21 with the Ags which are found to be opsonized with the complement fraction C3d facilitates grouping of the co-receptor with the BCR. The position of the CD21 allows the associated kinases to phosphorylate the tyrosine residues in the cytoplasmic domain of the CD19, and this binds to the tyrosine-kinases of the Src and the PI3-kinase family.

CO-STIMULATORY MOLECULES

Another important aspect in the activation of the B Cells is the presence of molecules which positively or negatively regulate the process. Together these are known as co-stimulatory molecules.

B cell activating factor (BAFF) is a cytokine and member of the TNF family. It is produced by a wide variety of cells (neutrophils, monocytes, macrophages, DCs, and T Cells) [24]. It is essential for the maturation and survival of the B Cells since it participates in the processes of differentiation and proliferation.

To date, three BAFF receptors have been identified:

i) BAFF-R

ii) TACI (transmembrane activator, calcium modulator, and cyclophilin ligand interactor)

iii) BCMA (B Cell maturation factor).

Interaction with the BAFF-R is the most critical to making maturation possible and causing BAFF-R to act in combination with the BCR . Elevated levels of BAFF have been observed in the sera of patients with SLE, Sjögren's Syndrome (SS), and rheumatoid arthritis (RA) [24].

i)   APRIL (A proliferation-inducing ligand)

It is a BAFF homologue that binds to TACI and BCMA but does not interact with BAFF-R. In addition to its co-stimulatory function, APRIL improves the ability of B Cells to present Ag and to increase their survival time and also regulates tolerance. On the other hand, it promotes the proliferation and survival of malignant B Cells and other tumoral cells. As for BAFF, elevated levels of APRIL have been observed in the sera of patients with SLE [25].

ii)   CD40

It is a transmembranal glycoprotein type I receptor, belongs to the TNF receptor superfamily. It is expressed on a great variety of cells (e.g., monocytes, Ag-presenting cells, endothelial cells, smooth muscle, fibroblasts, keratinocytes, and platelets) and in all the stages of the B Cells. This receptor N-terminal extracellular domain includes several cysteines, has four subregions, and binds to its ligand (CD40L or CD154) through the 2nd and 3rd subregion. The interaction between the CD40 and its ligand, which is present in the T Cells, increases the expression of cytokines (IL-2, IL-6, IL-10, TNF-α, Lymphotoxin-α, and TGF-β), chemokines, metalloproteinases of the matrix, growth factors, and adhesion molecules.

This allows signalling processes to occur through activation of several protein tyrosine kinases (PTK) such as ERK-1, ERK-2, p38, and JNK. This, permits the activation of several transcription factors such as NF-kB, AP-1, and NF-AT. These processes lead to maturation, differentiation, and cell proliferation of the B Cells with the subsequent production of Abs and, finally, the production of memory B Cells. Additionally, mutations in this molecule, or in its ligand, are responsible for the syndrome of hyper Ig M linked to chromosome X. Although this CD40-CD154 interaction mediates many mechanisms of the humoral and cell immune responses, it is also implicated in a wide spectrum of chronic inflammatory and autoimmune diseases. The blockage of this signaling route is therefore considered to be a potential therapeutic mechanism for these pathologies [26].

Other co-stimulatory molecules: the B Cell expresses another series of molecules from the super families CD28/B7 and TNF/TNFR which interact directly with the T Cells as co-stimulatory molecules. Included among these are B7-1 (CD80), B7-2 (CD86), CD70, the ICOS ligand (ICOS-L), the CD30 ligand (CD30-L or CD153), the 4-1BB ligand (4-1BBL), SLAM (CD150), etc [12].

MOLECULES OF ADHESION

B - cell mobilization requires adhesion mechanisms in which several types of molecules participate such as chemokines, their receptors, the selectins, and integrins.

Lymphoid chemokines are a group of chemokines/receptors that are expressed constitutively in the lymphoid tissue cells and aid in the recirculation of the lymphocytes. They include CXCL12, CXCL13, CCL19, CCL21, CXCR5, CCR7, and CXCR4 [27]. The differential positioning of the B Cells in the GC or in the external part of the follicles is regulated by the EBI2 receptor coupled to protein G (also known as GPR183) which directs the B Cells to the perifollicular and interfollicular areas. This location of the B Cells mediated by EBI2 is important for the first stages of the Ab response [27]. Molecules such as S1P (Sphingosine 1 Phosphate) and its S1PR1 receptor, in turn, control the exit of the B Cells from the lymph nodules [27]. The Ab-secretory cells express high levels of integrins such as α4β1 and LFA-1 as well as ICAM-1, α5β1, and α6β1.

The plasma cells in the intestine and the mammary glands express α4β7 [28,29]. The selectins are another family of molecules that contribute to the adhesion and mobilization of the B Cells. The plasmocytic have a high expression of PSGL-1 (P selectin glycol-protein ligand 1) which recognizes the P and the E selectin [28]. Another molecule that participates in the B Cell homing processes is the CD22, a member of the Siglec (sialic acid-binding immunoglobulin-like lectin) family which preferentially binds sugars with α2,6 -sialic acid radicals and is mainly present in mature B Cells [28].

B CELL SUBSETS

Mature B Cells can be divided into several subsets based on their location, cell surface phenotype, Ag specificity, and activation routes.

The transitional B Cells are considered to be the first stages of development of the B Cells once they leave the bone marrow to migrate to the secondary lymphoid organs. The lymphocytes CD20+, CD21±, CD23±, IgM++, and IgD± CD38++ are designated B Cell transitional type-1 (T1) and differentiate from type 2 (CD20+, CD21++, CD23±, IgM++, and IgD++ CD38±). The transitional B Cells T2 can evolve into marginal zone B Cells or GC [22,30,31].

The Follicular B Cells (FoB) or B-2. These are generated directly in the bone marrow and reach the follicles of secondary lymphoid organs and the circulation. They are considered to be resting (naive) cells and constitute the largest subpopulation of B Cells. Their differentiation is influenced by a great variety of factors including chemokines, BCR signalling, and some Ags. They participate in T-dependent (TD) immune responses since they can use the BCR to engulf the Ag, process it, and present it to the Ag-specific T Cells [32].

The Marginal zone B Cells (MZB).

This type of cell is located as a sentinel in the marginal zones of the spleen which correspond to the interphase between the circulation and the splenic lymphoid tissue. These B Cells also inhabit the inner wall of the subcapsular sinus of the lymph nodes, the epithelium of tonsillar crypts, and the subepithelial dome of intestinal Peyer's patches.

In humans, they present the following phenotype: IgM (high) IgD(low) CD1c+ CD21(high) CD23−CD27+. MZB express high levels of TLR (similar to macrophages, DCs, and granulocytes) phenomena that allow them to play a role of a bridge between innate and adaptive immune responses. MZB have the ability to rapidly respond to an Ag-specific stimulus by using both T-independent (TI) and dependent (TD) mechanisms and to transform into plasma cells that secrete IgM, IgG1, IgG2 (for both, TD and TI pathways), IgA1 (on the TD pathway), and IgA2 (on the TI pathway) low affinity Abs [33].

B1 B Cells

These are the first B Cells to form in the fetal liver. They subdivide into B1a and B1b with the former expressing the glycoprotein of membrane CD5, which is absent in the latter. Both express CD9 and CD45RA markers, are involved in type TI immune responses, are found in the peritoneal and pleural cavities, and are the main source of circulating Abs. As with the MZB, the B-1 responds rapidly to

Ag-specific stimuli and transforms into plasma cells. Their numbers have been observed to increase in experimental studies and in humans with autoimmune diseases.

Seven sub-populations of mature peripheral B Cells have been identified in human tonsils based on the expression of two surface markers (CD38 and IgD). This has made it possible for a TD model for the differentiation of mature B Cells to be proposed.

The subpopulations suggested are:

i)   B- cell mature naïve (Bm)

ii)   B- cell mature 1, Bm1 (CD38- IgD+)

iii)   Bm2 (CD38+ IgD+)

These three would be activated by their specific Ag in the extra-follicular areas through interaction with interdigital DC and Ag-specific T Cells. Once activated, the three can be transformed into Bm2' founder cells of GC (CD38++ IgD+), and then differentiate into Bm3 centroblasts (CD38+++ IgD-). These Bm3 cells are selected during their differentiation into Bm4 centrocytes (CD38++ IgD-) as a function of their BCR affinity. Finally, these cells differentiate into either memory B Cells (CD38+ IgD-), Bm5 cells (CD38-IgD-), or high affinity plasma cells.

Plasmocyte or Ab-secretory cells. These differentiate from an activated B Cell which, in the presence of IL-2 and IL-10, stops expressing surface molecules such as CD19, CD20, CD22, HLA class II molecules, and their BCR. These cells also lose the ability to divide. At the same time, they undergo a series of cellular modifications, e.g., an increase in their cytoplasm due to enhanced growth of the endoplasmic reticulum that is required to harbour the high number of ribosomes for robust production of Abs.

They also stop expressing CXCR5 and CXCR7 and increase CXCR4 which causes them to lose contact with the DC and forces the Tfh cells to migrate from the GC to the medullar cords of the ganglia [22].

Two classes of plasma cells are known: Short-lived cells, which are located in the medulla of the ganglia and, later, quickly exit to the circulation and seek the site where the Ag enter to initiate, in situ, the production of specific IgM type Abs. Long-lived cells migrate to a special niche in the bone marrow following the expression of SDF-1 by the stromal cells. Within this niche, an extended production of IgG type Abs, which can be used to mount a prolonged or permanent defence against the Ag that originally activated the B Cells, is initiated. The prolonged survival of these latter cells is due to the effect of IL-16. Development of short- or long-lived plasma cells depends on the expression of the transcription factor Blimp-1 (B lymphocyte-induced maturation protein-1) [22].

Memory B Cells. There are several subsets of memory B Cells that are classified based on their origin, the differential expression of CD27, and the isotype of the mIg being expressed.

Three different origins for the cells have been described: i) the spleen, ii) the germinal center, and iii) the intestine lamina propria outside the GC. In the spleen, they present CD27-IgG+ markers. At the GC, they are CD27+IgM+IgD- and change from mIg to CD27+IgG/IgA+. Last of all, those generated in the intestine express CD27-IgA+ [22,33].

Regulatory B Cells (Bregs). B Cells also liberate a wide variety of cytokines and, as with the T Cells, can be classified according to the profile of cytokines that they produce. Thus, the Bregs are a functional sub-set of B Cells, and they contribute to the maintenance of the fine equilibrium required to guarantee tolerance.

Bregs restrict the excessive inflammatory responses that are produced during autoimmune diseases or that can be caused by unresolved infections. IL-10 is fundamental to the function of Bregs since they inhibit pro-inflammatory cytokines (IFN-γ, IL-17), reduce the expression of the MHC clase II molecules and support the differentiation of Tregs [32]. It has also been reported that CD40-CD154 interaction is an essential activation pathway for the Bregs. With regard to the Breg surface markers, there is considerable controversy and the consensus is that there is no single marker, or even set of markers that make identification of this type of regulatory cell possible. Among the markers reported in these types of cells are: CD1dhigh, CD5+, CD19+, CD24high, CD27variable, CD38 variable, CD138 variable, Ig M (high), and IL-10+ [32].

INNATE B CELL HELPERS

It has also been demonstrated that B Cells receive additional help from other cells besides the T-helper cells. These include: the iNKT, DCs, epithelial cells, macrophages, and diverse granulocytes, including neutrophils, eosinophils, basophils, and mastocytes. The iNKT cells express a TCR invariant Vα14+ that recognizes soluble glycolipids, e.g., α-galactosylceramide, presented by DCs or sub-capsular macrophages in the CD1d context. Soluble glycolipids improve the expression of CD40L and IFN-α, which stimulates the maturation of DCs in the efficient antigen-presenting cells. These interact with the TFH cells to form active CGs with the consequent generation of long-living plasma cells that produce IgG [35,36].

 The B Cell helper neutrophils (Nbh) occupy the perimarginal zone of the spleen in the absence of inflammation or infection. They interact with perifollicular B Cells and MZB through the liberation of APRIL, BAFF, CD40L, IL-6, and IL-21 in response to stimuli by cytokines and microbial products. This interaction results in CSR processes by which the plasma cells generated stop expressing Ig M and start to produce IgG and IgA [34]. In general, we can say that these innate immune cells can stimulate and help the response of Abs to both TD and TI processes. For the former, these cells make use of helper signals for B Cells in the GC and in the central lymphoid sites such as the bone marrow. On top of this, the TI type responses take place on the surface of the mucosa and in the marginal zone of the spleen to give rise to a rapid response from natural Abs [32,33].

TYPES OF IMMUNE RESPONSES MEDIATED BY ABS

Traditionally, the humoral immune response mediated by Abs is classified based on whether or not the B Cells receive help from the T Cells, i.e., if they are TD or TI responses of the thymus [37]. One charactistic of the TD response is the induction of follicular GCs in which the Tfh cells select B Cells with high affinity BCRs by somatic mutation and cause them to differentiate into memory B – cells.

In contrast, the TI response may be provoked by microbial ligands, which are classified as type TI -1 or by extensive cross-linking of the BCR with the Ag, which is known as type TI -2 [37].

Recent studies describe the existence of two new mechanisms that participate in the B- cell response, e.g., the B Cells can also receive TD type help but from cells of innate immune system. Some examples are those induced from iNKT cells which are classified as TD - 2. Furthermore, an innate TI-3 type response has been described that involves myeloid cells such as B Cell helper neutrophils (NBH) [34], monocytes, eosinophils, mastocytes, and basophils [38].

Much remains to be discovered with regard to the steps in the human B - cell response, including which cells and molecules are involved in the new mechanisms described above.

B LYMPHOCYTES AND IMMUNOGLOBULINS INTERACTIONS

HISTORICAL PERSPECTIVE

- In the 1940s and 1950s, when antibodies were known as "antitoxins" and "antisera" and the immune response was primarily studied as a serum response to antigenic challenge (largely from deliberate immunization although to some extent from response to disease) it was sufficient to label them simply as "antibodies."

- It is important to remember that until the 1950s, there were few ways to partition serum proteins, and most relied on techniques that separated albumins from globulins (in medicine this became known as the A/G ratio).

- In the 1960s, once electrophoresis became commonplace, the globulins were divided into a 1, a 2, ß, and $_\gamma$? globulins. The connection between antibodies and $_\gamma$ globulins followed. "Sizing" columns were required to distinguish immunoglobulins into those that were "heavy" (IgM), "regular" (IgA, IgE, IgD, IgG), and "light" (light chain dimers).

- Only after immunoelectrophoresis was it clear that there were other "classes" of immunoglobulins.

- Finally, with the discovery of myeloma proteins as "gamma globulins" or "immunoglobulins," the clear class and subclass (isotype) distinctions that we know today became common place.

- When hybridomas and the immortalization of B cells became popular, further distinctions became evident [39].

STRUCTURE OF ANTIBODY

The immunoglobulin molecule is a complex structure of four polypeptide chains. The central structural component of the molecule is the Ig domain. The four-polypeptide chains are organized as a homodimer structure of a heterodimer between a heavy and light chain. Both chains contain variable and constant domains, with the heavy chain having two or three more constant domains than the light chain. Dimerization between the heavy and light chain variable domains and the first constant domain occurs as a result of hydrophobic interactions as well as a set of disulphide bonds at the carboxy-terminal end. A homodimer of this heavy–light chain configuration is then produced and held together by disulphide bonds in the hinge and tight hydrophobic interactions of the other constant domains. Therefore, an immunoglobulin contains two heavy chains (typically 55 kD each) and two light chains (25 feature of immunoglobulin structure[40].

By enzymatic and/or chemical cleavage, the immunoglobulin molecule can be broken into a number of "sections" or "fragments.". The Fab (fragment antigen binding) portion acquired in this cleavage would monovalent bind to antigen. Two of these regions are produced per immunoglobulin as cleavage occurs N terminal to the disulfide bonds of the hinge [41,42]. The remaining portion, the Fc (fragment crystallizable), was found to crystallize under low ionic conditions. Nisonoff et al.[43] and

Palmer and Nesenoff [44] found that pepsin cleavage produced the bivalent F(ab) 2 that upon exposure to reducing conditions could be separated into Fab monomeric units.

Properties of B-Cell Epitopes that are Determined by the Nature of the Antigen-Binding Site

Several generalizations have emerged from studies in which the molecular features of the epitope recognized by B cells have been established. The ability to function as a B-cell epitope is determined by the nature of the antigen-binding site on the antibody molecules displayed by B cells. Antibody binds to an epitope by weak non-covalent interactions, which operate only over short distances. For a strong bond, the antibody's binding site and the epitope must have complementary shapes that place the interacting groups near each other. This requirement poses some restriction on the properties of the epitope. The size of the epitope recognized by a B cell can be no larger than the size of the antibody's binding site. For any given antigen-antibody reaction, the shape of the epitope that can be recognized by the antibody is determined by the shape assumed by

A B cell antigen receptor is an antibody expressed on antigen reactive B cells that is similar to secreted antibody but is membrane-bound due to an extra domain at the Fc portion of the molecule. Upon antigen recognition by the membrane-bound immunoglobulin, noncovalently associated accessory molecules mediate transmembrane signalling to the B cell nucleus. The immunoglobulin and accessory molecule complex are similar in structure to the antigen receptor–CD3 complex of T lymphocytes. The cell surface membrane-bound immunoglobulin molecule serves as a receptor for antigen, together with two associated signal-transducing Igα/Igβ molecules

Igα and Igβ are proteins on the B cell surface that are noncovalently associated with cell surface IgM and IgD. They link the B cell antigen-receptor complex to intracellular tyrosine kinases. Anti-Ig binding leads to their phosphorylation. Igα and Igβ are required for expression of IgM and IgD on the B cell surface. Disulfide bonds link Igα and Igβ pairs that are associated noncovalently with the membrane Ig cytoplasmic tail to form the B cell receptor complex (BRC). The Igα and Igβ cytoplasmic domains bear immunoreceptor tyrosine-based activation motifs (ITAMs) that participate in early signalling when antigens activate B cells.

Igα/Igβ (CD79a/CD79b): The Igα/Igβ heterodimer interacts with immunoglobulin heavy chains for signal transduction. In the pro-B cell stage, rearrangement of the immunoglobulin heavy chain gene leads to expression of surface membrane immunoglobulin (mIgμ). mIgμ associates with Igα/Igβ and surrogate light chain in pre-B cells or ordinary light chains in B cells to form the precursor B cell receptor and B cell receptor, respectively. Igα and Igβ are expressed before immunoglobulin heavy chain gene rearrangement. They are products of mb-1 and B29 genes, respectively. Allelic exclusion is mediated through signal transduction via Igα and Igβ and depends on intact tyrosine residues.

Specificity refers to the recognition by an antibody or a lymphocyte receptor of a specific epitope in the presence of other epitopes for which the antigen-binding site of the antibody or of the lymphoid cell receptor is specific.

A B cell coreceptor is a three-protein complex that consists of CR2, TAPA-1, and CD19. CR2 unites not only with an activated component of complement, but also with CD23. TAPA-1 is a serpentine membrane protein. The cytoplasmic tail of CD 19 is the mechanism through which the complex interacts with lyn, a tyrosine kinase. Activation of the coreceptor by ligand binding leads to union of phosphatidyl inositol-3' kinase with CD19 resulting in activation. This produces intracellular signals that facilitate B cell receptor signal transduction.

TAPA-1 is a serpentine membrane protein that crosses the cell membrane four times. It is one of three proteins comprising the B cell coreceptor. It is also call CD81. CD19 is an antigen with a 90-kDa mol wt that has been shown to be a transmembrane polypeptide with at least two immunoglobulin-like domains.

The CD19 antigen is the most broadly expressed surface marker for B cells, appearing at the earliest stages of B cell differentiation. The CD19 antigen is expressed at all stages of B cell maturation, from the pro-B cell stage until just before the terminal differentiation to plasma cells. CD19 complexes with CD21 (CR2) and CD81 (TAPA-1). It is a coreceptor for B lymphocytes.

B cell markers that are used routinely for immunophenotyping by flow cytometry include CD19, CD20, and CD21.

CD20 is a B cell marker with a 33-, 35-, and 37-kDa mol wt that appears relatively late in the B cell maturation (after the pro-B cell stage) and then persists for some time before the plasma cell stage. Its molecular structure resembles that of a transmembrane ion channel. The gene is on chromosome 11 at band q12-q13. It may be involved in regulating B cell activation. CD21 (Figure 6.12) is an antigen with a 145-kDa mol wt, that is expressed on B cells and, even more strongly, on follicular dendritic cells. It appears when surface Ig is expressed after the pre-B cell stage and is lost during early stages of terminal B cell differentiation to the final plasma cell stage.

CD21 is coded for by a gene found on chromosome 1 at band q32. The antigen functions as a receptor for the C3d complement component and also for Epstein–Barr virus. CD21, together with CD19 and CD81, constitutes the co-receptor for B cells. It is also termed CR2. CD21 is a 145-kDa glycoprotein component of the B cell receptor. CD21 is a membrane molecule that participates in transmitting growth-promoting signals to the interior of the B cell. It is the receptor for the C3d fragment of the third component of complement, CR2. The CD21 antigen is a restricted B cell antigen expressed on mature B cells. It is present at high density on follicular dendritic cells (FDC), the accessory cells of the B zones. Also called complement receptor 2 (CR2).

CD22 is a molecule with an α130- and β140-kDa mol wt that is expressed in the cytoplasm of B cells of the pro-B and pre-B cell stage and on the cell surface on mature B cells with surface Ig. The antigen is lost shortly before the terminal plasma cell phase. The molecule has five extracellular immunoglobulin domains and shows homology with myelin adhesion glycoprotein and with N-CAM (CD56). It participates in B cell adhesion to monocytes and T cells. Also called BL-CAM.

A plasmablast is an immature cell of the plasma cell lineage that reveals distinctive, clumped nuclear chromatin developing endoplasmic reticulum and a Golgi apparatus. It is a B lymphocyte in a lymph node that is beginning to reveal plasma cell features. A plasmacyte is a plasma cell and are antibody producing cells. Immunoglobulins are present in their cytoplasm and secretion of immunoglobulin by plasma cells has been directly demonstrated in vitro. Increased levels of immunoglobulins in some pathologic conditions are associated with increased numbers of plasma cells, and conversely, their number at antibody-producing sites increases following immunization.

Plasma cells develop from B cells and are large spherical or ellipsoidal cells, 10 to 20 μm in size. Mature plasma cells have abundant cytoplasm, staining deep blue with Wright's stain, and have an eccentrically located round or oval nucleus, usually surrounded by a well-defined perinuclear clear zone. The nucleus contains coarse and clumped masses of chromatin, often arranged in a cartwheel fashion. The nuclei of normal, mature plasma cells have no nucleoli, but those of neoplastic plasma cells, such as those seen in multiple myeloma, have conspicuous nucleoli. The cytoplasm of normal plasma cells has conspicuous Golgi complex and rough endoplasmic reticulum and frequently contains vacuoles. The nuclear to cytoplasmic ratio is 1:2. By electron microscopy, plasma cells show very abundant endoplasmic reticulum, indicating extensive and active protein synthesis. Plasma cells do not express surface immunoglobulin or complement receptors, which distinguishes them from B lymphocytes. An example of plasma cell antigen is a murine plasmacyte membrane alloantigen. It may be designated PC-1, PC-2.

Pyroninophilic cells are cells whose cytoplasm stains red with methyl green pyronin stain. This signifies large quantities of RNA in the cytoplasm, indicating active protein synthesis. For example, plasma cells or other protein producing cells are pyroninophilic.

Antibody-secreting cells are differentiated B lymphocytes that synthesize the secretory form of immunoglobulin. Antibody-secreting cells result from antigen stimulation. They may be found in the lymph nodes, spleen, and bone marrow. A signal peptide is the leader sequence, a small sequence of amino acids that shepherds the heavy or light chain through the endoplasmic reticulum and is cleaved from the nascent chains prior to assembly of a completed immunoglobulin molecule [43].

ANTIGEN–ANTIBODY INTERACTIONS

Stimulation of B lymphoid cells by antigen leads to the formation of immunoglobulin molecules (antibodies), which may enter into a number of different types of immunological and chemical reactions.

These have been classified into (1) primary (2) secondary (3) tertiary reactions.

The primary reaction is the actual binding of antibody, via its Fab or antigen binding fragment, to its homologous antigen forming an antibody–antigen complex. After the two substances are brought into contact, their initial union takes place almost instantaneously (within milliseconds). Primary interaction refers to antigen and antibody binding that may or may not lead to a secondary visible reaction such as precipitation. Primary antigen–antibody interaction may be measured by equilibrium dialysis, the Farr assay, fluorescence polarization, fluorescence quenching, and selected radioimmunoassays such as radioimmunoelectrophoresis.

Antigen-binding capacity is determined by assay of the total capacity of antibody of all immunoglobulin classes to bind antigen. This refers to primary as opposed to secondary or tertiary manifestations of the antigen–antibody interaction. Equilibrium dialysis measures the antigen-binding capacity of antibodies with the homologous hapten, and the Farr test measures primary binding of protein antigens with the homologous antibody.

Secondary reactions are those visible effects resulting from antibody–antigen binding such as precipitation, agglutination, flocculation, complement fixation, and so on.

Tertiary reactions which may result from either primary or secondary interactions of antibody with antigen, include those in vivo biological manifestations of antibody reactivity. Some in vitro secondary interactions, such as cytophilic reactions (adherence of the antibody via its Fc to a cell surface) may, when occurring in vivo, give rise to tertiary manifestations. Because reactions occur in vivo, they tend to be very complex and are subject to many variables.

In an immune response, antibodies are directed against specific conformational areas on the antigen molecule referred to as antigenic determinants. Antigens are macromolecules which stimulate antibody production. Antibody populations directed against these macromolecules are notoriously heterogeneous with respect to their antibody specificity and affinity since antibodies to different antigenic determinants may be present simultaneously in the sera. Bivalent and multivalent antibodies directed against multi determinant antigens result in the formation of large antibody–antigen aggregates of the type (Ab) x (Ag) y varying in size, complexity, and solubility [43].

TUMOR IMMUNOLOGY

TERMINOLOGIES AND DEFINITION

NEOPLASM: neoplasm is any new and abnormal growth that may be either a benign or malignant tumor.

CANCER: It is an invasive, metastatic, and highly anaplastic cellular tumor that leads to death.

NEOANTIGENS: It includes tumor associated antigens. New antigenic determinants may also emerge when a protein changes conformation or when a molecule is split, exposing previously unexpressed epitopes.

CARCINOGEN: A carcinogen is any chemical or physical cancer-producing agent. Carcinogens comprise the epigenetic type that does not damage DNA but causes other physiological alterations that predispose to cancer, and the genotoxic type that reacts directly with DNA or with micromolecules that then react with DNA. A carcinoma is a malignant tumor composed of epithelial cells that infiltrate surrounding tissues and lead to metastases.

CHORIOCARCINOMA: A choriocarcinoma is an unusual malignant neoplasm of the placenta trophoblast cells in which the fetal neoplastic cells are allogeneic in the host. On rare occasions, these neoplasms have been "rejected" spontaneously by the host.

SARCOMAS: These tumors are arising from connective tissue.

BENIGN TUMOR: A benign tumor is an abnormal proliferation of cells that leads to a growth that is localized and contained within epithelial barriers. It does not usually lead to death, in contrast to a malignant tumor.

MALIGNANT TUMOR: is an adjective that means leading to death, as by a malignant neoplasm.

METASTASIS: is the transfer of disease from one organ or part to another not directly connected with it. For example, malignant tumors may need anatomical sites distant from the primary tumor's site of origin, leading to the establishment of secondary tumors.

MALIGNOLIPIN : (historical) is a substance claimed in the past to be specific for cancer and to be detectable in the patient's blood early in the course of the disease. This is no longer considered valid. Malignolipin is comprised of fatty acids, phosphoric acid choline, and spermine. When injected into experimental animals, it can produce profound anemia, leukopoiesis, and cachexia.

ONCOGENES: These genes are with the capacity to induce neoplastic transformation of cells.

PROTOONCOGENES

They are derived from either normal gene termed protooncogenes or from oncogenic RNA (oncorna) viruses. Their protein products are critical for regulation of gene expression or growth signal transduction. Translocation, gene amplification, and point mutation may lead to neoplastic transformation of protooncogene. Oncogenes may be revealed through use of viruses that induce tumors in animals or by derivation of tumor causing genes from cancer cells. There are more than 20 protooncogenes and cellular oncogenes in the human genome. An oncogene alone cannot produce cancer. It must be accompanied by malignant transformation which involves multiple genetic steps. Oncogenes encode four types of proteins that include growth factors, receptors, intracellular transducers, and nuclear transcription factors.

Proto-oncogenes are expressed during "regulated growth," such as embryogenesis, wound healing, regeneration of damaged liver, and stimulation of cell mitosis by growth factors. Proto-oncogenes are highly conserved, being detected in species as divergent as yeast, Drosophila, and humans. These genes encode for growth factors, growth factor receptors with tyrosine kinase activity, regulatory proteins in signal transduction, non-receptor tyrosine kinases, serine/threonine kinases, and transcription factors [44]. The encoded proteins play a crucial role in cellular growth, differentiation and in apoptosis or programmed cell death [45].

Viral oncogenes arise by recombination between cellular proto-oncogenes and the genome of non-transforming retroviruses. Proto-oncogenes can also be activated to cancer-causing oncogenes by mechanisms independent of retroviral involvement. These mechanisms include point mutations and gross DNA rearrangements such as translocation and gene amplification, and it is these mechanisms that generate the oncogenes observed in human and rodent tumors.

Tumor Antigens

The sub-discipline of tumor immunology involves the study of antigens on tumor cells and the immune response to these antigens.

Two types of tumor antigens have been identified on tumor cells: tumor-specific transplantation antigens (TSTAs) and tumor-associated transplantation antigens (TATAs).

Tumor-specific antigens are unique to tumor cells and do not occur on normal cells in the body. They may result from mutations in tumor cells that generate altered cellular proteins; cytosolic processing of these proteins would give rise to novel peptides that are presented with class I MHC molecules, inducing a cell-mediated response by tumor-specific CTLs.

Tumor-associated antigens, which are not unique to tumor cells, may be proteins that are expressed on normal cells during fetal development when the immune system is immature and unable to respond but that normally are not expressed in the adult. Reactivation of the embryonic genes that encode these proteins in tumor cells results in their expression on the fully differentiated tumor cells. Tumor-associated antigens may also be proteins that are normally expressed at extremely low levels on normal cells but are expressed at much higher levels on tumor cells.

It is now clear that the tumor antigens recognized by human T cells fall into one of four major categories:

- Antigens encoded by genes exclusively expressed by tumors

- Antigens encoded by variant forms of normal genes that have been altered by mutation

- Antigens normally expressed only at certain stages of differentiation or only by certain differentiation lineages

- Antigens that are over expressed in particular tumors

Many tumor antigens are cellular proteins that give rise to peptides presented with MHC molecules; typically, these antigens have been identified by their ability to induce the proliferation of antigen-specific CTLs or helper T cells

Tumor-Specific Antigens

Tumor-specific antigens have been identified on tumors induced with chemical or physical carcinogens and on some virally induced tumors. Demonstrating the presence of tumor-specific antigens on spontaneously occurring tumors is particularly difficult because the immune response to such tumors eliminates all of the tumor cells bearing sufficient numbers of the antigens and in this way selects for cells bearing low levels of the antigens.

CHEMICALLY OR PHYSICALLY INDUCED TUMOR ANTIGEN

Methylcholanthrene and ultraviolet light are two carcinogens that have been used extensively to generate lines of tumor cells. When syngeneic animals are injected with killed cells from a carcinogen-induced tumor-cell line, the animals develop a specific immunologic response that can protect against later challenge by live cells of the same line but not other tumor-cell lines .

Even when the same chemical carcinogen induces two separate tumors at different sites in the same animal, the tumor antigens are distinct and the immune response to one tumor does not protect against the other tumor. The tumor-specific transplantation antigens of chemically induced tumors have been difficult to characterize because they cannot be identified by induced antibodies but only by their T-cell–mediated rejection.

One experimental approach that has allowed identification of genes encoding some TSTAs. When a mouse tumorigenic cell line(tum+), which gives rise to progressively growing tumors, is treated in vitro with a chemical mutagen, some cells are mutated so that they no longer are capable of growing into a tumor.

Role of B-lymphocytes in tumor microenvironment

The role of B-lymphocyte in tumor-microenvironment is much less discussed or almost neglected for many reasons. Reconsidering the potentiality of B-lymphocyte, it could redefine the role of B-cell in tumor microenvironment. The role of B-lymphocyte is yet considered as a controversy by various authors and researchers. Surprisingly, both characteristic role of B-lymphocyte as pro-tumorogenic and anti-tumorogenic entity can be reconsidered to improvise our existing immunotherapeutic strategy [33]

THE ANTI-TUMOROGENIC RESPONSES OF B-LYMPHOCYTES

The anti-tumorogenic response of B-lymphocyte is mainly based production of tumor specific antibodies [46,47]. As in any other regular pathogenic infection it evokes the patient's innate immunity to resolve the infection by itself through recognition of antigen and producing antibodies against it. It is mediated through the pathway of Immunoglobulin G dependent antibody production [48]. IgG-mediated enhancement of the antibody response to soluble antigens is Complement dependent [49]. This is based on two types of experiments. First, enhancement of the B cell memory response by total Ig/antigen complexes was abolished in C3-depleted mice [50]. Second, IgG mAb of C-activating isotypes (IgG2,IgG2h) were more efficient enhancers than non-C-activating isotypes (IgA, IgGI).

However, the Ig/antigen-complexes used in the first study consisted of hyperimmune serum antibodies which were not separated into classes . It is therefore possible that the Complement dependency was due to IgM-containing complexes Thus, IgM and IgGh mAb (which generally are efficient C activators) as well as IgGl and IgA (which generally are poor C activators) sometimes do and sometimes do not enhance the complement pathway [51].And thereby, the body develops a permanent resistance towards the causative agent. The production of tumor antigen and tumor-associated antigen is also crucial for activating the immune system.

Normally, the Immunoglobulin G binding to bacteria makes it more visible for removing both the pathogenic organism and the toxic products secreted by it [52]. The potent cytotoxic function of Immunoglobulins can be therapeutically targeted to produce tumor-specific cytotoxic antibodies and enhance the tumor response of tumor. The evidence-based data obtained through clinical trial on human lymphoma patients, when treated with Rituximab, proved with a convincing evidence of FcYRs being involved in the therapeutic pathway [53].

Another study done in mice rendered B cell deficient by treatment with rabbit anti-mouse IgM (anti-mu) antibodies from birth fail to respond when primed with soluble protein antigens in CFA, as measured by T cell proliferation when challenged with antigen in vitro. The role of B cells in T cell priming in vivo was examined by adoptively transferring hapten-specific B cells into anti-mu mice, followed by immunization with haptenated Ag in CFA. The T cell proliferative response to OVA of anti-mu BALB/c mice was partially restored by the administration of TNP or FITC-specific B cells and immunization with TNP-OVA or FITC-OVA, respectively. This reconstitution was Ag-specific, inasmuch as hapten-binding B cells restored the T cell responses to OVA in mice immunized with the same hapten coupled to OVA. The mechanism of B cell reconstitution of T cell priming in anti-mu mice was addressed using parental to F1 B cell transfers. The Ia restriction pattern of the activated T cells from these mice indicated that both direct presentation of Ag by transferred B cells

28

and antibody-mediated enhancement of Ag presentation by non-B, host Ag-presenting cells occurred. Thus, Ag-specific B lymphocytes play a critical role in priming of T cells in vivo [54].

Tumor infiltrating B lymphocytes are considered as better APCs (Antigen presenting cells) of our immune system[53]. Activated B cells can serve as APCs for both CD4[+] and CD8[+] T cells, the prime advantage over the DCs dendritic cells is that it can selectively present cognate AG collected, through the surface Immunoglobulin molecules, even at minimal concentration of Ag [54]. However , DCs are considered essential for the initial T cell priming , whereas B cells may promote T cell expansion and memory formation [55-57] .Consistent with the findings of ovarian cancers it establishes the fact that lack of intra-tumoral DCs contain Tumor infiltrating B- lymphocytes (TIL-Bs) in close reaction with T cells . This establishes the complex and powerful interaction between both [55].

 B cells can also promote differentiation of Th1, Cytotoxic T-cell and can aid in T cell mediated immune response. The release of Granenzyme B can directly kill cancer cells and support the tumor suppressive actions of B-cells in tumor microenvironment [58]. Release of IFNα can stimulate TLR agoinst to kill tumor cells through the TRAIL signalling activity [59]. TRAIL Endogenous TRAIL is expressed as a 281–amino acid type II trans-membrane protein, which is anchored to the plasma membrane and presented on the cell surface. TRAIL was independently identified by Wiley and colleagues and Pitti and colleagues in 1995 and 1996, respectively, and sequence alignments indicated its close relation to other death ligands, with highest sequence similarities reported for Fas Ligand [60].

TRAIL is expressed by natural killer cells, which, following the establishment of cell–cell contacts, can induce TRAIL dependent apoptosis in target cells [61]. Physiologically, the TRAIL-signalling system was shown to be essential for immune surveillance, for shaping the immune system through regulating T-helper cell 1 versus T-helper cell 2 as well as "helpless" CD8þ T-cell numbers, and for the suppression of spontaneous tumor formation [61-63].

TRAIL-Induced Apoptosis Initiation: Signalling through Death and Decoy Receptors

TRAIL induces apoptosis through ligation with its cognate death receptors TRAIL-R1 (also known as DR4) and TRAIL-R2, and the trimerization of TRAIL around a central zinc atom via cysteine230 is essential for its apoptotic potential [64-65]. TRAIL binding is followed by receptor trimerization, and groups of trimerized death receptors can further cluster together to form bigger aggregates.

The intracellular death domains of the receptors and promote the recruitment and activation of initiator caspase8 within the death-inducing signalling complex. In most cells, caspase-8 then initiates apoptosis through Bid cleavage and the mitochondrial apoptosis pathway. Both the formation of the caspase-activating DISC, as well as the subsequent signalling network leading to apoptosis execution, can be modulated through a multitude of complex regulatory processes.

Additional TRAIL receptors, which are incapable of transducing the death signal because they lack a functional intracellular death domain, have been identified. A B C D. Simplified overview of TRAIL-mediated apoptosis signalling. A, trimers of TRAIL can bind to the extracellular regions of TRAIL-R1, TRAIL-R2, TRAIL-R3, and TRAIL-R4. The proapoptotic TRAIL-R1 and TRAIL-R2 comprise cytosolic regions, including a death domain (DD), which is missing in the antiapoptotic TRAIL-R3 and TRAIL-R4. TRAIL-R3 also lacks the transmembrane region [66].

Osteoprotegerin can serve as a soluble decoy receptor. B, antiapoptotic TRAIL-R3 forms homotrimers following TRAIL binding. TRAIL-R4 can also form heterotrimers with TRAIL-R1 and/or TRAIL-R2. These receptor clusters are unable to transduce the TRAIL signal further and, therefore, act as antiapoptotic TRAIL scavengers. C, TRAIL-R1 or TRAIL-R2 can recruit FADD to form the DISC. Procaspase-8 and cFLIP (a catalytically inactive caspase-8 homolog) compete for FADD binding via their death effector domains (DED). Procaspase-8 consists of a DED-containing prodomain, as well as large and small catalytic subunits. Heterodimers of caspase-8 and the long splice variant cFLIP have a very limited substrate repertoire and, in most cases, cannot transduce the apoptosis signal. The short splice variant of cFLIP (not shown) forms inactive heterodimers with caspase-8. D, induced

30

proximity of 2 procaspase-8 zymogens at the DISC results in autocatalytic cleavage of the linkers between the procaspase-8 subunits and caspase-8 activation. Active caspase-8 either resides at the DISC or, once fully processed, can be released into the cytosol. E, active caspase-8 cleaves Bid, inducing the mitochondrial apoptosis pathway, or directly activates effector caspase-3. XIAP suppresses caspase-9 and caspase-3 activity [67].

The receptors TRAIL-R3, TRAIL-R4, and osteoprotegerin [68]. TRAIL-R3 and TRAIL-R4 are alternatively also referred to as decoy receptors 1 and 2 (DcR1, DcR2). TRAIL-R4 (DcR2) bears huge similarities to TRAIL-R1 and TRAIL-R2; however, it contains only a truncated cytosolic death domain. TRAIL-R3 (DcR1) consists of an extracellular cysteine-rich structure that resembles the proapoptotic TRAIL receptors and is associated with the plasma membrane through a COOH terminal glycosyl-phosphatidylinositol anchor. It is still highly debated whether overexpression of TRAIL-R3 or TRAIL-R4 correlates with cellular apoptosis resistance upon TRAIL exposure, and high expression levels are rarely found naturally in isolated cancer cell lines.

The exact molecular details of how decoy receptors inhibit TRAIL-induced apoptosis in addition to their obvious role as TRAIL scavengers are not fully resolved and may differ between TRAIL-R3 and TRAIL-R4. For example, it was reported that TRAIL-R3 exclusively forms homotrimers upon TRAIL binding, whereas TRAIL-R4 may also aggregate into heterotrimers with activated TRAIL-R1 and TRAIL-R2. Such heterotrimers are incapable of forming a functional DISC required for apoptosis initiation. Relatively little is known about osteoprotegerin, the fifth receptor capable of TRAIL binding. Osteoprotegerin negatively regulates osteoclastogenesis and is largely secreted as a soluble protein that might act as a scavenger for soluble TRAIL [69]. Uncertainties remain about the molecular mechanisms of death and decoy receptor interaction, and it remains to be conclusively shown whether the relative abundance of death versus decoy receptors could serve to indicate cellular susceptibility to TRAIL-induced apoptosis. Notably, these were however not approved in murine prostate cancer study[70]

Pro-tumorogenic responses of B-cell

On the other hand, the pro-tumorogenic responses include the production of various cytokines and interleukins especially IL 35, TGF-β and IL- 10, that aids in tumor progression. The various B-cell regulatory subtypes also promote metastasis through the activation of various angiogenic and pro-inflammatory factors. Secretion of IL-8 an endothelial growth factor can promote angiogenesis and tumor growth [71]. The presence of chemokine CXCL-13 is closely contributed as a factor for tumor progression along with various lymphotoxins such as STAT3, NF-κβ [72]. Evidence of bladder metastasis holds determinable in the role played by b-cells in metastasis of tumor progression to various sites of the body [73]. The study demonstrated that infiltrating B cells could enhance Bladder carcinoma invasion and metastasis *via* modulation of IL-8/AR/MMPs signals. Future studies could develop an effective therapeutic strategy to interrupt these newly identified B cells/IL-8/AR/MMPs signals to better suppress metastasis.

Activity of IL-8

Interleukin-8 (IL-8) is a proinflammatory CXC chemokine associated with the promotion of neutrophil chemotaxis and degranulation. This chemokine activates multiple intracellular signalling pathways downstream of two cell-surface, G protein coupled receptors (CXCR1and CXCR2). Interleukin-8 (IL-8), alternatively known as CXCL8, is a proinflammatory CXC chemokine. Transcription of the IL8 gene encodes for a protein of 99 amino acids that is subsequently processed to yield a signalling competent protein of either 77 amino acids in non-immune cells or 72 amino acids in monocytes and macrophages. Increased expression of IL-8 and/or its receptors has been characterized in cancer cells, endothelial cells, infiltrating neutrophils, and tumor-associated macrophages, suggesting that IL-8 may function as a significant regulatory factor within the tumor microenvironment.

The induction of IL-8 signalling activates multiple upstream signalling pathways :

a)   impinge on gene expression via regulation of numerous transcription factor activities

b)   modulate the cellular proteome at the level of translation

c)   effect the organization of the cell cytoskeleton through posttranslational regulation of regulatory proteins.

As a consequence of the diversity of effectors and downstream targets, IL-8 signalling promotes angiogenic responses in endothelial cells, increases proliferation and survival of endothelial and cancer cells, and potentiates the migration of cancer cells, endothelial cells, and infiltrating neutrophils at the tumor site. Accordingly, IL-8 expression correlates with the angiogenesis, tumorigenicity, and metastasis of tumors in numerous xenografts and orthotopic in vivo models. Recently, IL-8 signalling has been implicated in regulating the transcriptional activity of the androgen receptor, underpinning the transition to an androgen independent proliferation of prostate cancer cells. In addition, stress and drug-induced IL-8 signalling has been shown to confer chemotherapeutic resistance in cancer cells. Therefore, inhibiting the effects of IL-8 signalling may be a significant therapeutic intervention in targeting the tumor microenvironment [73].

The tumor induced proliferation of B-cells can directly have a role in regulatory activity of myeloid derived suppressor cells (MDSCs) suppresses the cytotoxic activity of T- cells by down-regulation the production of CD4+aand CD8 + cells. Tumor B regulatory lymphocytes are also closely associated with the activity of TGFβ which suppresses the anti-tumor response through the up-regulating activity of ROS and NO production [74].Activated B cells and Bregs are known to upregulate and use TGFb, for example, in conversion of FoxP3þ T cells and modulation of macrophages [75,76]. Similarly, we recently reported that murine and human tBregs also convert FoxP3þ T cells by overexpressing TGFb [77-89].Using various complementary in vitro and in vivo modeling studies, it demonstrate that tBregs and cancer-induced B cells also use the TGFb-TgfbR1/2 axis in the activation (education) of both Mo and PMN subsets of cancer-expanded MDSC.

Studies conducted in mice with implanted murine mammary tumor demonstrates association of B cells with recruitment and proliferation of T regulatory cells and reduced recruitment of CD49 + and

33

CD8 $^+$ CTLs (cytotoxic T lymphocytes) within the tumor microenvironment. First, the presence of TGFb neutralizing but not control, Ab was sufficient to inhibit the MDSC education in vitro.

Second, the blocked TgfbR1 signalling with a specific inhibitor SB431542 during the education of mMT-MDSC with tBregs, we failed to detect the upregulation of ROS production and suppression of T cells.

As a result, these MDSC supported metastasis less efficiently in mMT mice upon their adoptive transfer. Similarly, the TgfbR1 inhibitor also blocked the education of human MDSC by tBregs induced by CM of MDA-MB-231 cells and tBreg-like cells of patients with B-CLL. confirmed these results using MDSC from tumor-bearing mice with myeloid cells deficient in TgfbR2, which is required for the signalling of TgfbR1 [80]. Unlike mMT-MDSC, tBregs failed to educate MDSC with TgfbR2 KO, as shown by the loss of upregulation of ROS production, T-cell inhibition, and ability to support metastasis upon transfer into mMT mice.

Thus, these results unequivocally indicate that cancer-induced B cells and tBregs render the full regulatory function of MDSC by, at least, targeting their TgfbR1/ TgfbR2 signalling axis. In support, others recently reported that 4T1 cancer also fails to metastasize in BALB/c mice deficient in TgfbR2 in myeloid cells [81], suggesting that this is due to the inability of their MDSC to get education from tBregs.

B cells play an important role in adaptive immune response is widely recognised through pan markers of CD 19 and CD 20 [82]. However, the heterogeneity in B-cell function doesn't appeal both for its pro-tumorogenic or anti-tumorogenic responses. Therefore, the clinical information and standardisation of immune based staining methods and procedures are to be standardised t establishing the role of B-lymphocytic activity in tumor microenvironment from studies conducted prior would be a due necessary to start with. The immune-escape of a tumor through the PD-1/PD-L1 (programmed cell death-1 / programmed cell death ligand -1) activity is also to be critically recommended to be discussed in reverse the immune escape mechanism of tumors and improve anticancer immune responses [83-85].

The PD-1 (programmed cell death-1) receptor is expressed on the surface of activated T cells. Its ligands, PD-L1 and PD-L2, are expressed on the surface of dendritic cells or macrophages. PD-1 and PD-L1/PD-L2 belong to the family of immune checkpoint proteins that act as co-inhibitory factors that can halt or limit the development of the T cell response. The PD-1/PD-L1 interaction ensures that the immune system is activated only at the appropriate time in order to minimize the possibility of chronic autoimmune inflammation [86].

The role of PD-1/PD-L1 in cancer

Under normal conditions, the immune system performs a series of steps which lead to an anticancer immune response and cancer cell death, known as the cancer immunity cycle [87]:

1. Tumor cells produce mutated antigens that are captured by dendritic cells
2. The dendritic cells prime T cell with tumor antigen and stimulate the activation of cytotoxic T cells
3. Activated T cells then travel to the tumor and infiltrate the tumor environment
4. The activated T cells recognize and bind to the cancer cells
5. The bound effector T cells release cytotoxins, which induce apoptosis in their target cancer cells

The PD-1/PD-L1 pathway represents an adaptive immune resistance mechanism exerted by tumor cells in response to endogenous immune anti-tumor activity. PD-L1 is over expressed on tumor cells or on non-transformed cells in the tumor microenvironment [88]. PD-L1 expressed on the tumor cells binds to PD-1 receptors on the activated T cells, which leads to the inhibition of the cytotoxic T cells. These deactivated T cells remain inhibited in the tumor microenvironment.

Using PD-1/PD-L1 and immunotherapy

Monoclonal antibody therapies against PD-1 and PD-L1 are being routinely used including:

--

- Nivolumab, an anti-PD-1 drug developed by Bristol-Myers Squibb, which is approved for previously treated metastatic melanoma and squamous non-small cell lung cancer.
- Pembrolizumab, developed by Merck is approved for previously treated metastatic melanoma. There are several other immunotherapy options being used or in development.

Combination immunotherapy

The efficiency of the immune checkpoint blockade with monoclonal antibodies in cancer treatment is remarkable, but not all patients respond to a single therapy. To enhance and broaden the anti-tumor activity of immune checkpoint inhibition the next step is combining agents with synergistic mechanisms of action. An example of this is the success of the combination of PD-1/PD-L1 inhibition blockage with complementary checkpoint inhibitor CTLA-4 in melanoma and non-small cell lung cancer [89].

A study conducted to understand the clinicopathologic implication of mi-197 and PD-L1 analysed the number of recruited TILs and the correlation with various clinicopathologic features and prognosis in OSCC patients [90]. MicroRNAs (miRNAs) and long noncoding RNAs (lncRNAs) are important noncoding RNAs (ncRNAs), which display a remarkable variety of biological functions. ncRNAs can be classified by length (small, 18–200 nt; long, >200 nt) or by function (housekeeping ncRNAs and regulatory ncRNAs) [91], with research over the last two decades largely focusing on regulatory ncRNAs. miRNAs, which are ~22 nt long, are the most widely studied class of regulatory ncRNAs, and these molecules mediate post-transcriptional gene silencing in animals by controlling the translation of mRNAs into proteins [92]. lncRNAs, longer than 200 nt, are another subtype of regulatory ncRNAs that have a broad repertoire of functions in chromatin modification as well as in transcriptional, post-transcriptional, and translational regulation [93,94].

miRNAs and lncRNAs are expressed at different levels in multiple cell and tissue types; they are also involved in tumorigenesis and the progression of aggressive cancer phenotypes [95].These molecules are identified as either carcinogenetic or carcinostatic; are associated with cell growth, proliferation, migration, invasion, and apoptosis; and can even alter immune functions. RNA sequencing has confirmed that miRNA and lncRNA profiles can serve as highly sensitive and specific diagnostic and prognostic biomarkers [96-100]. Because these molecules can be detected in diverse tumor tissues compared to normal samples and are associated with different clinicopathologic characteristics, differentially expressed miRNAs and lncRNAs can be employed to assess the pathogenesis of diseases, including non-small-cell lung cancer (NSCLC), gastric cancer (GC), colorectal cancer (CRC), and melanoma, as well as clinical prognosis [101-102].

Recent studies of miRNAs and lncRNAs have indicated their latent therapeutic value for successful clinical translation. Results have confirmed that miRNAs and lncRNAs function as crucial regulators in different drug therapies, including chemotherapy, immunotherapy, and targeted molecular therapy, and the associated mechanisms have been investigated.

miRNAs and lncRNAs Participate in Chemotherapy

Although chemotherapy remains a mainstay of anticancer treatment, the multi-organ toxicity and chemoresistance associated with this treatment strategy continues to be problematic.

Accumulating evidence shows that ncRNAs have an important role in cellular sensitivity to chemotherapy due to their specific regulatory features [103].

The significance of miRNAs in anticancer chemotherapy has been demonstrated by multiple studies, and the associated mechanisms include regulation of different targets [104]. For example, miR-197, miR-130b, and lncRNA MALAT1 confer cisplatin resistance in NSCLC by targeting the signal transducer and activator of transcription 3 (STAT3) and Wnt/β-catenin pathways, and lncRNA TP53TG1 enhances cellular sensitivity through the miR-18a/PTEN axis [105-108].1

In contrast, miR-125a-5p and lncRNA TUSC7 are able to reverse cisplatin resistance in oesophageal squamous cell carcinoma (ESCC) by reducing the levels of STAT3 and miR-224, respectively [109-110]. miR-503 and miR-623 inhibit resistance to different drugs by regulating cyclin D1-3 (CCND1-3) and targeting Bcl-2, miR-374b-5p and miR-15 were found to enhance the chemosensitivity of cancer cells by modulating apoptotic pathways [111-113].

miRNAs are small RNA molecules binding to partially complementary sites in the 3'-UTR of target transcripts and repressing their expression. miRNAs orchestrate multiple cellular functions and play critical roles in cell differentiation and cancer development. The study analyzed miRNA profiles in B-cell subsets during peripheral B-cell differentiation as well as indiffuse large B-cell lymphoma (DLBCL) cells. Our results show temporal changes in the miRNA expression during B-cell differentiation with a highly unique miRNA profile in germinal center (GC) lymphocytes. We provide experimental evidence that these changes may be physiologically relevant by demonstrating that GC enriched hsa-miR-125b down-regulates the expression of IRF4 and PRDM1/ BLIMP1, and memory B cell–enriched hsa-miR-223 down-regulates the expression of LMO2.

It further demonstrate that although an important component of the biology of a malignant cell is inherited from its non-transformed cellular progenitor—GC centroblasts—aberrant miRNA expression is acquired upon cell transformation. A 9-miRNA signature was identified that could precisely differentiate the 2 major subtypes of DLBCL. Finally, expression of some of the miRNAs in this signature is correlated with clinical outcome of uniformly treated DLBCL patients [114].

Therefore, researches carried out to determine the actual functionality of B-lymphocyte in tumor microenvironment is highly critical and recommended. There is a need in identifying the pro-tumorogenic B cell markers to elucidate a criterion in isolating them and separating them within in the tumor microenvironment. Identifying the genes of tumors associated with immune –resistance and suppressing them through targeted therapy can also be considered at a genetic level study. The selective knocking off pro-tumorogenic responses of tumor can also be an integral part of genetic work up study. It may help in switching of cancer susceptibility from an immune-resistant to an immune susceptible state. In turn can be a possible way out for the most favourable outcome desired in immunotherapy protocols.

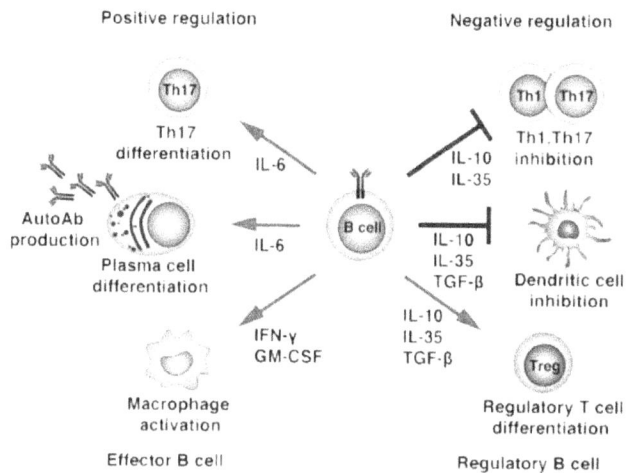

APPLIED ASPECTS OF B-LYMPHOCYTES IN IMMUNOTHERAPY

CD40 B-LYMPHOCYTES BASED VACCINES

Illustration of Biagi E, Rousseau R, Yvon E, Schwartz M, Dotti G, Foster A, Havlik-Cooper D, Grilley B, Gee A, Baker K, Carrum G, being the first clinical trial cancer vaccine that used CD 40 cells as cellular adjuvant in cancer regression therapy [115]. This involved vaccine contained transduced autologous leukemic B cells isolated from patients diagnosed with chronic lymphocytic leukaemia (CLL) combined with an adenoviral vector that contained human CD 40L gene were administrated to 9 patients. Out of which three patients demonstrated with positive results through 50% reduction in size of lymph node. Unfortunately, the drawback of the study was that the study induced T-cell response could not extend over the long term tumor –induced suppression. This study was the first ever favourable proof in implementing B-cell based immunotherapy and its role played in generating an antitumor response through activation of T-cells directly

Dendritic Cell Based PSMA Immunotherapy Using a CD40-Targeted Adenovirus Vector
Human prostate tumor vaccine and gene therapy trials using *ex vivo* methods to prime dendritic cells (DCs) with prostate specific membrane antigen (PSMA) have been somewhat successful, but to date the lengthy *ex vivo* manipulation of DCs has limited the widespread clinical utility of this approach. The study goal was to improve upon cancer vaccination with tumor antigens by delivering PSMA *via* a CD40-targeted adenovirus vector directly to DCs as an efficient means for activation and antigen presentation to T-cells. To test the approach, developed a mouse model of prostate cancer by generating clonal derivatives of the mouse RM-1 prostate cancer cell line expressing human PSMA (RM-1-PSMA cells). To maximize antigen presentation in target cells, both MHC class I and TAP protein expression was induced in RM-1 cells by transduction with an Ad vector expressing interferon-gamma (*Ad5-IFNγ*). Administering DCs infected *ex vivo* with CD40-targeted *Ad5-huPSMA*, as well as direct intraperitoneal injection of the vector, resulted in high levels of tumor-specific CTL responses against RM-1-PSMA cells pretreated with *Ad5-IFNγ* as target cells. CD40 targeting significantly improved the therapeutic antitumor efficacy of *Ad5-huPSMA* encoding PSMA when combined with *Ad5-IFNγ* in the RM-1-PSMA model. These results suggest that a CD-targeted adenovirus delivering PSMA may be effective clinically for prostate cancer immunotherapy [116].

Anti-CD40 mAb in development

The therapeutic anti-human CD40 mAbs Dacetuzumab and Lucatumumab are recombinant antibodies and have become the leading drug candidates in relation to antiCD40 based immunotherapy. Dacetuzumab is a humanized anti-CD40 agonistic mAb which triggers CD40-mediated signaling in various cells. Lucatumumab is a fully humanized antagonistic antibody against CD40 and exerts its primary function through opsonization followed by antibody-dependent cell-mediated cytotoxicity (ADCC) [117-119]. Administration of anti-CD40 mAb is most commonly systemically, e.g. by i.v. administration, but in some cases injection directly into the tumor has been tested and may result in a better therapeutic response[120] as demonstrated by, e.g. Fransen et al. It has been postulated, that a part of this beneficial effect is due to a slow release of the mAb which may prolong access for effector cells and at the same time reduce antibody-mediated side-effects and toxicity [121].

Dacetuzumab – the agonistic effect

The "first in man" clinical trial that tested the anti-CD40 agonistic antibody CP-870,893 (Kd of 0.4nmol/L) was described by Vonderheide et al.in 2007 [122]. The CP-870,893 mAb was tested in 15 patients with late stage melanoma and 14 patients with stages III and IV solid tumors of various types and a partial response was observed in four out of 15 melanoma patients but no response was observed in patients with other tumors. Since CP-870,893 is of the immunoglobulin (Ig)G2 isotype, it is unlikely that ADCC occurred27 and it was therefore believed that the primary effect of the therapy was associated with unspecific stimulation of effector cells from the immune system, and TNF-a and IL-6 were indeed elevated in serum.

Lucatumumab – the antagonistic effect

Lucatumumab, also known as CHIR 12.12 or HCD122, is a fully humanized recombinant mAb of the IgG1 isotype which targets human CD40. Lucatumumab is a potent antagonist and has a high binding affinity for CD40 (Kd 0.5nmol/L). It is able to mediate the killing and clearance of tumor cells via ADCC and other opsonization mechanisms.

In a study by Tai et al., the authors demonstrated that CHIR12.12 was able to bind to CD40+ MM cells from480% of MM patients. It was shown that CHIR-12.12 alone neither stimulated nor inhibited the CD40+ patients' myeloma cells, and was able to block the CD40L-induced growth and survival signals without altering the constitutive MM proliferation.

Furthermore, the treatment-inhibited myeloma cell adhesion to fibronectin and bone marrow stromal cells (BMSCs), indicating a reduced capacity for local spreading. The antagonistic activity was biochemically confirmed by immunoblotting studies in which CHIR-12.12 was shown to down-regulate the CD40L-induced phosphorylation of AKT, nuclear factor kappa-light-chain-enhancer of activated B cells (NF-kB), and extracellular signal-regulated kinases (ERK) in MM cells. Moreover, CHIR-12.12 antagonized CD40Linduced secretion of IL-6 and vascular endothelial growth factors (VEGF) in both MM cells and BMSCs, a mechanism that may reduce tumor angiogenesis. Finally, the authors were able to demonstrate ADCC activity of CHIR-12.12 against CD40-expressing myeloma cells2after treatment [123].

Tremelimumab

Tremelimumab is a fully human anti-cytotoxic T lymphocyte-associated antigen-4 (CTLA-4) monoclonal antibody, which blocks the binding of CTLA-4 to B7.1 or B7.2 on APCs, leading to enhanced T cell activation and inhibition of Treg responses. In a phase I study, Tremelimumab has been shown to induce antitumor responses in patients with metastatic melanoma47. Currently, the drug is being testing in a study named "Tremelimumab and CP-870,893 in Patients with Metastatic Melanoma". The rationale behind this study is that by utilizing two different antibodies, which target inducing and inhibitory immune mechanisms and/or controls the tumor growth by different mechanisms, the overall response of the combined therapy will be a greater reduction of tumor cells in patients with metastatic melanoma. The patients received Tremelimumab and CD40 agonist mAb CP-870.893 i.v. over 30min on day 2, 22, 43, and 64. In the absence of disease progression and unacceptable toxicity, the treatment was repeated every 12 weeks for four courses. The trial is still recruiting participants [124].

The goal of immunotherapy is to activate the immune system in a specific way in order to increase recognition and killing of the cancer cells. In immunotherapy, different therapies including cytokines, cancer vaccines, cell therapies (adoptive T cell transfer and DC-based vaccination), and antibodies are used to activate the immune system in either

a direct or an indirect manner. Some forms of immunotherapy, e.g. cytokine therapy and antibody therapy, are already an integrated part of cancer treatments. For example, a-interferon (Introna) and IL-2 (Proleukin) are used against malignant melanoma and renal cancer. The antibody-based therapies include Bevacizumab (Avastin) and Cetuximab (Erbitux) for the treatment of colon-cancer, and the antibody Rituximab (MabThera) for the treatment of lymph node cancer. It may be of interest to test the combination of such therapies with anti-CD40 targeting in the future. Indeed, an increasing number of possible combination therapies is arising [125]. Several other types of therapies including surgery, chemotherapy, and radiation therapy have been applied clinically [126-130]. It may indeed be of interest to test the combination of such with CD40 targeting also. Depending on the cancer type, different combination therapies have been tested. For the treatment of CLL, the purine analog fludarabine has been investigated with other chemotherapy agents, e.g. cyclophosphamide which have shown promising outcomes [130-133]. Furthermore, the results from a chemo-immunotherapy study consisting of fludarabine, cyclophosphamide, and the chimeric monoclonal antibody Rituximab showed a high CR rate in previously untreated CLL65 and are of interest to combine with antiCD40 treatment.

EXPERIMENTAL STUDIES DONE

CD20+ Tumor Infiltrating B Lymphocyte in Oral Squamous Cell Carcinoma: Correlation with Clinicopathologic Characteristics and Heat Shock Protein 70 Expression

In an immunohistochemical study of 50 OSCC patients which was conducted to evaluate the relationship between tumor infiltrating B-lymphocyte and HSP70 expression in OSCC, the expression of CD20+ was present evidently in cases of oral squamous cell carcinoma. Positive staining of B-lymphocytes infiltrated cells were highly evident in OSCCs with the molecular staining technique. The data analysis showed significant correlation between peritumoral CD20+ B-lymphocyte infiltration and lymph node metastasis with P = 0.047. The relationship between markers and clinicopathologic data was evaluated using Mann-Whitney test, Chi-square test, logistic regression model and Spearman's correlation coefficient. Thus, the study concluded with expression of both CD20+ B-lymphocyte and HSP70 in OSCC, both were considered as prognostic indicators. The evaluation of B-cells as therapeutic targets in OSCC patients was also recommended [134].

In a cohort study, of feline oral squamous cell carcinoma (OSCC) that shared clinical characteristics with head and neck squamous cell carcinoma (HNSCC) an immunohistochemistry marker study was conducted to study the B-cell and T-cell infiltration, in which intratumoral B-cell infiltrates were detected within tumor stroma by IHC staining for CD79a and CD20, along with T-cell subsets of CD4 (Tregs) by fork head transcription factor (FoxP3) involving both neoplastic epithelium and stroma of patient biopsies. 92% of the cases, there was marked expression of CD20+ B-lymphocyte in tumor cells along with T-cell subsets of the Treg series and COX-2. The study assessed the role of immune response in the control of cancer. The statistical analysis performed using GraphPad Software Inc,.San Diego CA), and unpaired t-test was used to compare the different groups of cohorts. B-cell infiltrate scores and staining based on CD20 and CD79a were also compared separately. Thus, the study was a preliminary step to establish the relationship between immune markers shared by feline OSCC patients and human HNSCC[135].

In a study, that was conducted to analyse the tumor-infiltrating lymphocytes (TILs) in oral squamous cell carcinoma (OSCC), the evidence of tumor-specific immune response evoked by both T- and B-cells within the tumor were considered useful to develop immune-related therapies for oral cancer. The role of TIL-Bs, B-cells was first selected among others and were performed using anti-human CD20 microbeads and sorted using a PCR plate. The immunohistochemistry of the tumor cells showed dense cluster of CD20+ B lymphocytic cells which were mainly distributed along the follicle. The study observed that the density of T-cells was significantly greater than that of B-cells and was assessed using students test (p <0.001) in the intra-tumoral region. The study provided some insight towards the role of TILs in immune microenvironment of tumor to develop immune-related therapies[136].

In a study, conducted to analyse B-cell subsets in head and neck squamous cell carcinoma(HNSCC); B-cell subsets were analysed in HNSCC(n=38), non-cancerous mucosa(n=14) and peripheral blood from HNSCC(n=38) patients and healthy controls(n=20) by flow cytometry. The percentage of B-cells (CD19+/CD20+) were significantly higher in HPV+ HNSCC (1.13 ± 1.72%) compared to HPV- HNSCC (0.017 ± 0.33%; p = 0.024). The proportions of B-cells among live cells in the TME of early stage versus advanced stage was also similar (0.61 ± 1.44 % vs 0.34 ± 0.63%). The presence of CD20+ B-cells in the tumor microenvironment (TME) had been mainly linked to good prognosis and potential benefit in immune modulatory treatment options[137].

In an analytical cross-sectional study, performed on 53 human tongue tissues diagnosed histopathological as hyperkeratosis (11 cases), mild dysplasia (9 cases), moderate and severe dysplasia (14 cases) and squamous cell carcinoma (19 cases) and additionally 30 cases of parotid gland diagnosed as pleomorphic (14 cases) and carcinoma ex-pleomorphic adenoma(16 cases) was done to analyse the mononuclear cell infiltration. The Formalin-fixed, paraffin-embedded tissue sections initially stained with haematoxylin and eosin, and then primary antihuman antibodies against CD4, CD8, CD14, CD19+20, HLA/DR, p53 DAKO were used for immunohistochemical staining . The results suggested that the mean staining of four markers were more significant in Discoid Lupus

Erythematous and Lichen Planus lesions than in normal skin and that there was an increased

tendency of mature immune cells, especially of B-cells to infiltrate into malignant epithelial lesions.

A significant proportion of B-cells was found in hyperkeratosis and mild dysplastic lesions compared

with moderate and severe dysplasia and squamous cell carcinoma lesions (p=0.004)[138].

REFERENCES

1.   Markopoulos AK. Current aspects on oral squamous cell carcinoma. The open dentistry

journal. 2012; 6:126.

2.   Kumar V, Abbas AK, Aster JC. Robbins basic pathology e-book. Elsevier Health Sciences; 2017

Mar 8.

3.   Medler TR, Cotechini T, Coussens LM. Immune response to cancer therapy: mounting an

effective antitumor response and mechanisms of resistance. Trends in cancer. 2015 Sep 1;1(1):66-

75.

4.   Zoete, V. et al. (2013) Structure-based, rational design of T cell receptors. Front. Immunol.

268

5.   Linnemann, C. et al. (2014) TCR repertoires of intratumoral T-cell subsets. Immunol. Rev.

257, 72–82

6.   Gros, A. et al. (2014) PD-1 identifies the patient-specific CD8+ tumor-reactive repertoire

infiltrating human tumors. J. Clin. Invest. 124, 2246–2259

7.   Gubin, M.M. et al. (2014) Checkpoint blockade cancer immuno-therapy targets tumour-

specific mutant antigens. Nature 515, 577–581

8.   Beatty, G.L. et al. (2011) CD40 agonists alter tumor stroma and show efficacy against

pancreatic carcinoma in mice and humans. Science 331, 1612–1616

9.   Dushyanthen, S., Beavis, P.A., Savas, P. *et al.* Relevance of tumor-infiltrating lymphocytes in breast cancer. *BMC Med* **13,** 202 (2015).

10.   Cano RL, Lopera HD. Introduction to T and B lymphocytes. In Autoimmunity: From Bench to Bedside [Internet] 2013 Jul 18. El Rosario University Press.

11.   Nagasawa T. Microenvironmental niches in the bone marrow required for B Cell development. Nat Rev Immunol. 2006;6:107-16.

12.   Kurosaki T. B-lymphocyte biology. Immunol Rev. 2010;237:5-9. 44. Pieper K, Grimbacher B, Eibel H. B Cell biology and development. J Allergy Clin Immunol. 2013;131:959-71.

13.   Cruickshank MN, Ulgiati D. The role of notch signaling in the development of a normal B Cell repertoire. Immunol Cell Biol. 2010;88:117-24.

14.   Herzog S, Reth M, Jumaa H. Regulation of B Cell proliferation and differentiation by pre-B Cell receptor signalling. Nat Rev Immunol. 2009;9:195-205.

15.   Townsend MJ, Monroe JG, Chan AC. B Cell targeted therapies in human autoimmune diseases: an updated perspective. Immunol Rev. 2010;237:264-83

16.   Shlomchik MJ, Weisel F. Germinal center selection and the development of memory B and plasma cells. Immunol Rev. 2012;247:52-63.

17.   Cerutti A, Cols M, Puga I. Marginal zone B cells: virtues of innate-like antibody-producing lymphocytes. Nat Rev Immunol. 2013;13:118-32

18.   Macias-Perez IM, Flinn IW. B Cell receptor pathobiology and targeting in NHL. Curr Oncol Rep. 2012;14:411-8.

19.   http://www.cellsignal.com/ reference/pathway/B_Cell_Antigen.html

20.   Macias-Perez IM, Flinn IW. B Cell receptor pathobiology and targeting in NHL. Curr Oncol Rep. 2012;14:411-8.

21.   Choi MY, Kipps TJ. Inhibitors of B Cell receptor signaling for patients with B Cell malignancies. Cancer J. 2012;18:404-10.

22.   Pieper K, Grimbacher B, Eibel H. B Cell biology and development. J Allergy Clin Immunol. 2013;131:959-71.

23.   Weinstein E, Peeva E, Putterman C, Diamond B. B Cell biology. Rheum Dis Clin North Am. 2004;30:159-74

24.   Townsend MJ, Monroe JG, Chan AC. B Cell targeted therapies in human autoimmune diseases: an updated perspective. Immunol Rev. 2010;237:264-83.

25.   Dillon SR, Gross JA, Ansell SM, Novak AJ. An APRIL to remember: novel TNF ligands as therapeutic targets. Nat Drug Rev Discov. 2006;5:235-46.

26.   Chatzigeorgiou A, Lyberi M, Chatzilymperis G, Nezos A, Kamper E. CD40/CD40L signaling and its implication in health and disease. Biofactors. 2009;35:474-83.

27.   Girard JP, Moussion C, Forster R. HEVs, lymphatics and homeostatic immune cell trafficking in lymph nodes. Nat Rev Immunol. 2012;12:762-73.

28.   Cyster JG. Homing of antibody secreting cells. Immunol Rev. 2003;194:48-60. 60.

29.   Severinson E, Westerberg L. Regulation of adhesion and motility in B lymphocytes. Scand J Immunol. 2003;58:139-44

30.   Sims GP, Ettinger R, Shirota Y, Yarboro CH, Illei GG, Lipsky PE. Identification and characterization of circulating human transitional B cells. Blood. 2005;105:4390-8.

31.   Cornec D, Devauchelle-Pensec V, Tobon GJ, Pers JO, JousseJoulin S, Saraux A. B cells in Sjogren's syndrome: from pathophysiology to diagnosis and treatment. J Autoimmun. 2012;39:161-7.

32.   Pillai S, Cariappa A. The follicular versus marginal zone B lymphocyte cell fate decision. Nat Rev Immunol. 2009;9:767-77

33.   Cerutti A, Cols M, Puga I. Marginal zone B cells: virtues of innate-like antibody-producing lymphocytes. Nat Rev Immunol. 2013;13:118-32.

34.   Puga I, Cols M, Barra CM, et al. B cell-helper neutrophils stimulate the diversification and production of immunoglobulin in the marginal zone of the spleen. Nat Immunol. 2012;13:170-80.

35.   Cerutti A, Cols M, Puga I. Activation of B cells by non-canonical helper signals. EMBO Rep. 2012;13:798-810. 67.

36.   Cerutti A, Puga I, Cols M. New helping friends for B cells. Eur J Immunol. 2012;42:1956-68.

37.   Lange H, Zemlin M, Tanasa RI, et al. Thymus-independent type 2 antigen induces a long-term IgG-related network memory. Mol Immunol. 2008;45:2847-60.

38.   Vinuesa CG, Chang PP. Innate B cell helpers reveal novel types of antibody responses. Nat Immunol. 2013;14:119-26.

39.   Paul WE. MD ed. Fundamental immunology,. 1993:242.

40.   Hill RL, Delaney R, Fellows RE, et al. The evolutionary origins of the immunoglobulins. Proc Natl Acad Sci USA 1966;56:1762–1769.

41.   Plaut AG, Wistar R Jr, Capra JD. Differential susceptibility of human IgA immunoglobulins to streptococcal IgA protease. J Clin Invest 1974;54:1295–1300.

42.   Plaut AG, Gilbert JV, Artenstein MS, et al. Neisseria gonorrhoeae and neisseria meningitidis: extracellular enzyme cleaves human immunoglobulin A. Science 1975;190:1103–1105.

43.   Parish LC. Historical Atlas of Immunology, JM Cruse, RE Lewis, Taylor & Francis, New York (2005), 338 pp.

44.   Anderson MW, Reynolds SH, You M, Maronpot RM. Role of proto-oncogene activation in carcinogenesis. Environmental health perspectives. 1992 Nov;98:13-24.

45.   Hockenbery, D., Nunez, G., Milliman, C., Schreiber, R. D., and Korsmeyer, S. J. Preventing cell suicide: a new role for oncogenes. Nature 348: 334 (1990).

46.   Li Q, Lao X, Pan Q, Ning N, Yet J, Xu Y, et al. Adoptive transfer of tumor reactive B cells confers host T-cell immunity and tumor regression. Clin Cancer Res. 2011 Aug;17(15):4987–95.

47.   Eckert AW, Wickenhauser C, Salins PC, Kappler M, Bukur J, Seliger B. Clinical relevance of the tumor microenvironment and immune escape of oral squamous cell carcinoma. Journal of translational medicine. 2016 Dec;14(1):85.

48.   Nimmerjahn F. Molecular and cellular pathways of immunoglobulin G activity in vivo. ISRN Immunology. 2014 Mar 5;2014.

49.   Wiersma EJ, Nose M, Heyman B. Evidence of IgG-mediated enhancement of the antibody response in vivo without complement activation via the classical pathway. European journal of immunology. 1990 Dec;20(12):2585-9.

50.   E. Mossner, P. Br ̈unker, S. Moser et al., "Increasing the efficacy ̈ of CD20 antibody therapy through the engineering of a new type II anti-CD20 antibody with enhanced direct and immune effector cell—mediated B-cell cytotoxicity," Blood, vol. 115, no. 22, pp. 4393–4402, 2010.

51.   Klaus, G. G. B., Immunology 1978. 34: 643

52.   S. H. Lim, S. A. Beers, R. R. French, P. W. M. Johnson, M. J. Glennie, and M. S. Cragg, "Anti-CD20 monoclonal antibodies: historical and future perspectives," Haematologica, vol. 95, no. 1, pp. 135–143, 2010

53.   Nelson BH. CD20+ B cells: the other tumor-infiltrating lymphocytes. The Journal of Immunology. 2010 Nov 1;185(9):4977-82.

54.   Kurt-Jones, E. A., D. Liano, K. A. HayGlass, B. Benacerraf, M. S. Sy, and A. K. Abbas. 1988. The role of antigen-presenting B cells in T cell priming in vivo. Studies of B cell-deficient mice. J. Immunol. 140: 3773–3778.

55.   Tobon, G. J., Izquierdo, J. H. & Canas, C. A. B lymphocytes: development, tolerance, and their role in autoimmunity-focus on systemic lupus erythematosus. Autoimmune Dis. 2013, 827254 (2013)

56.   Milne, K., M. Ko¨bel, S. E. Kalloger, R. O. Barnes, D. Gao, C. B. Gilks, P. H. Watson, and B. H. Nelson. 2009. Systematic analysis of immune infiltrates in high-grade serous ovarian cancer reveals CD20, FoxP3 and TIA-1 as positive prognostic factors. PLoS ONE 4: e6412.

57.   Rodrı´guez-Pinto, D. 2005. B cells as antigen presenting cells. Cell. Immunol. 238: 67–75

58.   Wakim, L. M., J. Waithman, N. van Rooijen, W. R. Heath, and F. R. Carbone. 2008. Dendritic cell-induced memory T cell activation in nonlymphoid tissues. Science 319: 198–202

59.   Lundy, S. K. 2009. Killer B lymphocytes: the evidence and the potential. Inflamm. Res. In press.

60.   SmythMJ,CretneyE,TakedaK,WiltroutRH,SedgerLM,KayagakiN,   etal.Tumornecrosisfactor-relatedapoptosis-inducingligand(TRAIL) contributes to interferon gamma-dependent natural killer cell protection from tumor metastasis. J Exp Med 2001;193:661–70.

61.   8. Cretney E, Takeda K, Yagita H, Glaccum M, Peschon JJ, Smyth MJ. Increased susceptibility to tumor initiation and metastasis in TNFrelated apoptosis-inducing ligand-deficient mice. J Immunol 2002; 168:1356–61.

62.   9. JanssenEM,DroinNM,LemmensEE,PinkoskiMJ,BensingerSJ,Ehst BD, et al. CD4þT-cell help controls CD8þT-cell memory via TRAILmediated activation-induced cell death. Nature 2005;434:88–93.

63.   10. Zhang XR, Zhang LY, Devadas S, Li L, Keegan AD, Shi YF. Reciprocal expression of TRAIL and CD95L in Th1 and Th2 cells: role of apoptosis in T helper subset differentiation. Cell Death Differ 2003; 10:203–10.

64.   BodmerJL,MeierP,TschoppJ,SchneiderP.Cysteine230isessential forthestructureandactivityofthecytotoxicligandTRAIL.JBiolChem 2000;275:20632–7.

65.   HymowitzSG,O'ConnellMP,UltschMH,HurstA,TotpalK,Ashkenazi A, etal. A unique zinc-binding site revealed by a high-resolution X-ray structure of homotrimeric Apo2L/TRAIL. Biochemistry 2000;39: 633–40.

66.   Song JH, Tse MC, Bellail A, Phuphanich S, Khuri F, Kneteman NM, et al. Lipid rafts and nonrafts mediate tumor necrosis factor related apoptosis-inducing ligand induced apoptotic and nonapoptotic signals in non small cell lung carcinoma cells. Cancer Res 2007;67: 6946–55.

67.   Bin L, Thorburn J, Thomas LR, Clark PE, Humphreys R, Thorburn A. Tumor-derived mutations in the TRAIL receptor DR5 inhibit TRAIL signaling through the DR4 receptor by competing for ligand binding. J Biol Chem 2007;282:28189–94.

68.   Pennarun B, Meijer A,de Vries EG,Kleibeuker JH, Kruyt F, de Jong S. Playing the DISC: turning on TRAIL death receptor-mediated apoptosis in cancer. Biochim Biophys Acta 2010;1805:123–40.

69.   EmeryJG,McDonnellP,BurkeMB,DeenKC,LynS,SilvermanC,etal. Osteoprotegerin is a receptor for the cytotoxic ligand TRAIL. J Biol Chem 1998;273:14363–7.

70.   Ammirante M, Luo JL, Grivennikov S, Nedospasov S, Karin M. B-cell-derived lymphotoxin promotes castration-resistant prostate cancer. Nature. 2010 Mar;464(7286):302-5.

71.   Bindea, G. et al. (2013) Spatiotemporal dynamics of intratumoral immune cells reveal the immune landscape in human cancer. Immunity 39, 782–795 41.

72.   Luo JL, Tan W, Ricono JM, Korchynskyi O, Zhang M, Gonias SL, Cheresh DA, Karin M. Nuclear cytokine-activated IKKα controls prostate cancer metastasis by repressing Maspin. Nature. 2007 Apr;446(7136):690-4.

73.   Waugh DJ, Wilson C. The interleukin-8 pathway in cancer. Clinical cancer research. 2008 Nov 1;14(21):6735-41.

74.   Lund FE. Cytokine-producing B lymphocytes—key regulators of immunity. Current opinion in immunology. 2008 Jun 1;20(3):332-8.

75.   Bao Y, Cao X. The immune potential and immunopathology of cytokineproducing B cell subsets: A comprehensive review. J Autoimmun 2014; 55:10–23.

76.   Reyes JL, Wang A, Fernando MR, Graepel R, Leung G, van Rooijen N, et al. Splenic B cells from Hymenolepis diminuta-infected mice ameliorate colitis independent of T cells and via cooperation with macrophages. J Immunol 2015;194:364–78

77.   Olkhanud PB, Damdinsuren B, Bodogai M, Gress RE, Sen R, Wejksza K, et al. Tumor-evoked regulatory B cells promote breast cancer metastasis by converting resting CD4þ T cells to T-regulatory cells. Cancer Res 2011;71: 3505–15.

78.   Bodogai M, Lee Chang C, Wejksza K, Lai J, Merino M, Wersto RP, et al. AntiCD20 antibody promotes cancer escape via enrichment of tumor-evoked regulatory B cells expressing low levels of CD20 and CD137L. Cancer Res 2013;73:2127–38.

79.   Lee-Chang C, Bodogai M, Martin-Montalvo A, Wejksza K, Sanghvi M, Moaddel R, et al. Inhibition of breast cancer metastasis by resveratrolmediated inactivatio

80.   Taylor AW. Review of the activation of TGF-beta in immunity. J Leukoc Biol 2009;85:29–33

81.   Pang Y, Gara SK, Achyut BR, Li Z, Yan HH, Day CP, et al. TGF-beta signaling in myeloid cells is required for tumor metastasis. Cancer Discov 2013; 3:936–51.

82.   Lund FE. Cytokine-producing B lymphocytes—key regulators of immunity. Current opinion in immunology. 2008 Jun 1;20(3):332-8.

83.   Zhang, Y. et al. (2013) B lymphocyte inhibition of anti-tumor response depends on expansion of Treg but is independent of B-cell IL-10 secretion. Cancer Immunol. Immunother. 62, 87–99

84.   Tobon, G. J., Izquierdo, J. H. & Canas, C. A. B lymphocytes: development, tolerance, and their role in autoimmunity-focus on systemic lupus erythematosus. Autoimmune Dis. 2013, 827254 (2013).

85.   Xie M, Ma L, Xu T, Pan Y, Wang Q, Wei Y, Shu Y. Potential regulatory roles of microRNAs and long noncoding RNAs in anticancer therapies. Molecular Therapy-Nucleic Acids. 2018 Dec 7;13:233-43.

86. Barclay J, Creswell J, León J. Cancer immunotherapy and the PD-1/PD-L1 checkpoint pathway. Archivos espanoles de urologia. 2018 May;71(4):393-9

87. Chen, D. and Mellman, I. Oncology meets immunology: the cancer-immunity cycle. *Immunity* **39**, 1–10 (2013).

88. Pardoll, D.M. The blockade of immune checkpoints in cancer immunotherapy. *Nat Rev Cancer*, **12**, 252–264 (2012).

89. Ott, P.A., et al. (2017). Combination immunotherapy: a road map. *J Immunother Cancer*, **5**:16 (2017)

90. Ahn H, Yang JM, Kim H, Chung JH, Ahn SH, Jeong WJ, Paik JH. Clinicopathologic implications of the miR-197/PD-L1 axis in oral squamous cell carcinoma. Oncotarget. 2017 Sep 12;8(39):66178.

91. Cech TR, Steitz JA. The noncoding RNA revolution—trashing old rules to forge new ones. Cell. 2014 Mar 27;157(1):77-94.

92. Glasgow AM, De Santi C, Greene CM. Non-coding RNA in cystic fibrosis. Biochemical Society Transactions. 2018 Jun 19;46(3):619-30.

93. Ma P, Pan Y, Li W, Sun C, Liu J, Xu T, Shu Y. Extracellular vesicles-mediated noncoding RNAs transfer in cancer. Journal of hematology & oncology. 2017 Dec;10(1):57.

94. Tang S, Tan G, Jiang X, Han P, Zhai B, Dong X, Qiao H, Jiang H, Sun X. An artificial lncRNA targeting multiple miRNAs overcomes sorafenib resistance in hepatocellular carcinoma cells. Oncotarget. 2016 Nov 8;7(45):73257.

95. Mohr AM, Mott JL. Overview of microRNA biology. InSeminars in liver disease 2015 Feb (Vol. 35, No. 01, pp. 003-011). Thieme Medical Publishers.

96. Li ZH, Li L, Kang LP, Wang Y. Micro RNA-92a promotes tumor growth and suppresses immune function through activation of MAPK/ERK signaling pathway by inhibiting PTEN in mice bearing U14 cervical cancer. Cancer medicine. 2018 Jul;7(7):3118-31.

97.   Li C, Du X, Xia S, Chen L. MicroRNA-150 inhibits the proliferation and metastasis potential of colorectal cancer cells by targeting iASPP. Oncology reports. 2018 Jul 1;40(1):252-60.

98.   Ma P, Pan Y, Li W, Sun C, Liu J, Xu T, Shu Y. Extracellular vesicles-mediated noncoding RNAs transfer in cancer. Journal of hematology & oncology. 2017 Dec;10(1):57.

99.   Wang L, Wang F, Na L, Yu J, Huang L, Meng ZQ, Chen Z, Chen H, Ming LL, Hua YQ. LncRNA AB209630 inhibits gemcitabine resistance cell proliferation by regulating PI3K/AKT signaling in pancreatic ductal adenocarcinoma. Cancer Biomarkers. 2018 Jan 1;22(1):169-74.

100.   Yang X, Song JH, Cheng Y, Wu W, Bhagat T, Yu Y, Abraham JM, Ibrahim S, Ravich W, Roland BC, Khashab M. Long non-coding RNA HNF1A-AS1 regulates proliferation and migration in oesophageal adenocarcinoma cells. Gut. 2014 Jun 1;63(6):881-90.

101.   Ding X, Zhang S, Li X, Feng C, Huang Q, Wang S, Wang S, Xia W, Yang F, Yin R, Xu L. Profiling expression of coding genes, long noncoding RNA, and circular RNA in lung adenocarcinoma by ribosomal RNA-depleted RNA sequencing. FEBS Open Bio. 2018 Apr;8(4):544-55.

102.   Yang H, Wang S, Kang YJ, Wang C, Xu Y, Zhang Y, Jiang Z. Long non-coding RNA SNHG1 predicts a poor prognosis and promotes colon cancer tumorigenesis. Oncology reports. 2018 Jul 1;40(1):261-71.

103.   Sonawane VK, Mahajan UB, Shinde SD, Chatterjee S, Chaudhari SS, Bhangale HA, Ojha S, Goyal SN, Kundu CN, Patil CR. A chemosensitizer drug: Disulfiram prevents doxorubicin-induced cardiac dysfunction and oxidative stress in rats. Cardiovascular toxicology. 2018 Oct 1;18(5):459-70.

104.   Riquelme I, Letelier P, Riffo-Campos AL, Brebi P, Roa JC. Emerging role of miRNAs in the drug resistance of gastric cancer. International journal of molecular sciences. 2016 Mar;17(3):424.

105.   Fujita Y, Yagishita S, Hagiwara K, Yoshioka Y, Kosaka N, Takeshita F, Fujiwara T, Tsuta K, Nokihara H, Tamura T, Asamura H. The clinical relevance of the miR-197/CKS1B/STAT3-mediated PD-L1 network in chemoresistant non-small-cell lung cancer. Molecular therapy. 2015 Apr 1;23(4):717-27.

106. Zhang Q, Zhang B, Sun L, Yan Q, Zhang Y, Zhang Z, Su Y, Wang C. MicroRNA-130b targets PTEN to induce resistance to cisplatin in lung cancer cells by activating Wnt/β-catenin pathway. Cell biochemistry and function. 2018 Jun;36(4):194-202.

107. Fang Z, Chen W, Yuan Z, Liu X, Jiang H. LncRNA-MALAT1 contributes to the cisplatin-resistance of lung cancer by upregulating MRP1 and MDR1 via STAT3 activation. Biomedicine & Pharmacotherapy. 2018 May 1;101:536-42.

108. Xiao H, Liu Y, Liang P, Wang B, Tan H, Zhang Y, Gao X, Gao J. TP53TG1 enhances cisplatin sensitivity of non-small cell lung cancer cells through regulating miR-18a/PTEN axis. Cell & bioscience. 2018 Dec;8(1):23.

109. Zhao Y, Ma K, Yang S, Zhang X, Wang F, Zhang X, Liu H, Fan Q. MicroRNA-125a-5p enhances the sensitivity of esophageal squamous cell carcinoma cells to cisplatin by suppressing the activation of the STAT3 signaling pathway. International journal of oncology. 2018 Aug 1;53(2):644-58.

110. Chang ZW, Jia YX, Zhang WJ, Song LJ, Gao M, Li MJ, Zhao RH, Li J, Zhong YL, Sun QZ, Qin YR. LncRNA-TUSC7/miR-224 affected chemotherapy resistance of esophageal squamous cell carcinoma by competitively regulating DESC1. Journal of Experimental & Clinical Cancer Research. 2018 Dec;37(1):56.

111. Bovy N, Blomme B, Frères P, Dederen S, Nivelles O, Lion M, Carnet O, Martial JA, Noël A, Thiry M, Jérusalem G. Endothelial exosomes contribute to the antitumor response during breast cancer neoadjuvant chemotherapy via microRNA transfer. Oncotarget. 2015 Apr 30;6(12):10253.

112. Jiang L, Yang W, Bian W, Yang H, Wu X, Li Y, Feng W, Liu X. microRNA-623 targets cyclin D1 to inhibit cell proliferation and enhance the chemosensitivity of cells to 5-fluorouracil in gastric cancer. Oncology Research Featuring Preclinical and Clinical Cancer Therapeutics. 2018 Dec 27;27(1):19-27.

113.   Sun D, Wang X, Sui G, Chen S, Yu M, Zhang P. Downregulation of miR-374b-5p promotes chemotherapeutic resistance in pancreatic cancer by upregulating multiple anti-apoptotic proteins. International journal of oncology. 2018 May 1;52(5):1491-503.

114.   Malumbres R, Sarosiek KA, Cubedo E, Ruiz JW, Jiang X, Gascoyne RD, Tibshirani R, Lossos IS. Differentiation stage–specific expression of microRNAs in B lymphocytes and diffuse large B-cell lymphomas. Blood, The Journal of the American Society of Hematology. 2009 Apr 16;113(16):3754-64.

115.   Biagi E, Rousseau R, Yvon E, Schwartz M, Dotti G, Foster A, Havlik-Cooper D, Grilley B, Gee A, Baker K, Carrum G. Responses to human CD40 ligand/human interleukin-2 autologous cell vaccine in patients with B-cell chronic lymphocytic leukemia. Clinical cancer research. 2005 Oct 1;11(19):6916-23.

116.   Williams BJ, Bhatia S, Adams LK, Boling S, Carroll JL, Li XL, Rogers DL, Korokhov N, Kovesdi I, Pereboev AV, Curiel DT. Dendritic cell based PSMA immunotherapy for prostate cancer using a CD40-targeted adenovirus vector. PloS one. 2012;7(10).

117.   Byrd JC, Kipps TJ, Flinn IW, et al. Phase I study of the anti-CD40 humanized monoclonal antibody lucatumumab (HCD122) in relapsed chronic lymphocytic leukemia. Leuk Lymphoma 2012; 53:424–429

118.   Tai YT, Li X, Tong X, et al. Human anti-CD40 antagonist antibody triggers significant antitumor activity against human multiple myeloma. Cancer Res 2005;65:5898–5906.

119.   Advani R, Forero-Torres A, Furman RR, et al. Phase I study of the humanized anti-CD40 monoclonal antibody dacetuzumab in refractory or recurrent non-Hodgkin's lymphoma. J Clin Oncol 2009;27: 4371–4377.

120.   Jackaman C, Nelson DJ. Intratumoral interleukin-2/agonist CD40 antibody drives CD4+-independent resolution of treated-tumors and CD4+-dependent systemic and memory responses. Cancer Immunol Immunother 2012;61:549–560.

121.   Fransen MF, Sluijter M, Morreau H, et al. Local activation of CD8 T cells and systemic tumor eradication without toxicity via slow release and local delivery of agonistic CD40 antibody. Clin Cancer Res 2011;17:2270–2280.

122.   Vonderheide RH, Flaherty KT, Khalil M, et al. Clinical activity and immune modulation in cancer patients treated with CP-870,893, a novel CD40 agonist monoclonal antibody. J Clin Oncol 2007;25: 876–883.

123.   Tai YT, Li X, Tong X, et al. Human anti-CD40 antagonist antibody triggers significant antitumor activity against human multiple myeloma. Cancer Res 2005;65:5898–5906.

124.   Reuben JM, Lee BN, Li C, et al. Biologic and immunomodulatory events after CTLA-4 blockade with ticilimumab in patients with advanced malignant melanoma. Cancer 2006;106:2437–2444.

125.   Scott AM, Wolchok JD, Old LJ. Antibody therapy of cancer. Nat Rev Cancer 2012;12:278–287.

126.   Bell DJ, Wilson MW. Choroidal melanoma: natural history and management options. Cancer Control 2004;11:296–303.

127.   58. Cowey CL. Profile of tivozanib and its potential for the treatment of advanced renal cell carcinoma. Drug Des Devel Ther 2013; 7: 519–527.

128.   Fisher B. Biological research in the evolution of cancer surgery: a personal perspective. Cancer Res 2008;68:10007–10020.

129.   Hillmen P, Skotnicki AB, Robak T, et al. Alemtuzumab compared with chlorambucil as first-line therapy for chronic lymphocytic leukemia. J Clin Oncol 2007;25:5616–5623.

130.   Rai KR, Peterson BL, Appelbaum FR, et al. Fludarabine compared with chlorambucil as primary therapy for chronic lymphocytic leukemia. N Engl J Med 2000;343:1750–1757.

131.   Johnson S, Smith AG, Loffler H, et al. Multicentre prospective randomised trial of fludarabine versus cyclophosphamide, doxorubicin, and prednisone (CAP) for treatment of advanced-stage chronic lymphocytic leukaemia. The French Cooperative Group on CLL. Lancet 1996;347:1432–1438.

132.   Eichhorst BF, Busch R, Hopfinger G, et al. Fludarabine plus cyclophosphamide versus fludarabine alone in first-line therapy of younger patients with chronic lymphocytic leukemia. Blood 2006; 107:885–891.

133.   Flinn IW, Neuberg DS, Grever MR, et al. Phase III trial of fludarabine plus cyclophosphamide compared with fludarabine for patients with previously untreated chronic lymphocytic leukemia: US Intergroup Trial E2997. J Clin Oncol 2007;25:793–798.

134.   Taghavi N, Mohsenifar Z, Baghban AA, Arjomandkhah A. CD20+ tumor infiltrating b lymphocyte in oral squamous cell carcinoma: correlation with clinicopathologic characteristics and heat shock protein 70 expression. Pathology research international. 2018;2018.

135.   65. Keating MJ, O'Brien S, Albitar M, et al. Early results of a chemoimmunotherapy regimen of fludarabine, cyclophosphamide, and rituximab as initial therapy for chronic lymphocytic leukemia. J Clin Oncol 2005;23:4079–4088.

136.   DOI: 10.3109/08923973.2014.890626 Anti-CD40-mediated cancer immunotherapy 103
137.   Immunopharmacology and Immunotoxicology Downloaded from informahealthcare.com by Gazi Univ. on 12/30/14 For personal use only.

Additional references

1.   Beatty GL, Torigian DA, Chiorean EG, et al. A phase I study of an agonist CD40 monoclonal antibody (CP-870,893) in combination with gemcitabine in patients with advanced pancreatic ductal adenocarcinoma. Clin Cancer Res 2013;19:6286–6295.

2.   Vonderheide RH, Burg JM, Mick R, et al. Phase I study of the CD40 agonist antibody CP-870,893 combined with carboplatin and paclitaxel in patients with advanced solid tumors. Oncoimmunology 2013;2:e23033.

3.   Bensinger W, Maziarz RT, Jagannath S, et al. A phase 1 study of lucatumumab, a fully human anti-CD40 antagonist monoclonal antibody administered intravenously to patients with relapsed or refractory multiple myeloma. Br J Haematol 2012;159: 58–66.

4.   Van LS, Goyvaerts C, Maenhout S, et al. Preclinical evaluation of TriMix and antigen mRNA-based antitumor therapy. Cancer Res 2012;72:1661–1671.

5.   Jellinger KA, Attems J (2003) Incidence of cerebrovascular lesions in Alzheimer's disease: a post-mortem study. Acta Neuropathol 105:14-17.

6.   Keck S, Nitsch R, Grune T, Ulrich O (2003) Proteasome inhibition by paired helical filament-tau in brains of patients with Alzheimer's disease. J Neurochem 85:15-22.

7.   Hagn, M., E. Schwesinger, V. Ebel, K. Sontheimer, J. Maier, T. Beyer, T. Syrovets, Y. Laumonnier, D. Fabricius, T. Simmet, and B. Jahrsdo¨rfer. 2009. Human B cells secrete granzyme B when recognizing viral antigens in the context of the acute phase cytokine IL-21. J. Immunol. 183: 1838–1845

8.   Kemp, T. J., J. M. Moore, and T. S. Griffith. 2004. Human B cells express functional TRAIL/Apo-2 ligand after CpG-containing oligodeoxynucleotide stimulation. J. Immunol. 173: 892–899. 78. Ammirante, M., J. L. Luo, S. Grivennikov, S. Nedospasov, and M. Karin. 2010. B-cell-derived lymphotoxin promotes castration-resistant prostate cancer. Nature 464: 302–305.

9.   Bindea, G. et al. (2013) Spatiotemporal dynamics of intratumoral immune cells reveal the immune landscape in human cancer. Immunity 39, 782–795 41.

10.   Bindea, G. et al. (2014) The immune landscape of human tumors: implications for cancer immunotherapy. Oncoimmunology 3, e27456 42.

11.   Gu-Trantien, C. et al. (2013) CD4+ follicular helper T cell infiltration predicts breast cancer survival. J. Clin. Invest. 123, 2873–2892

12.   Teng, M.W.L. et al. (2015) From mice to humans: developments in cancer immunoediting. J. Clin. Invest. 125, 3338–3346

13.   Ammirante M, Luo JL, Grivennikov S, Nedospasov S, Karin M. B-cell-derived lymphotoxin promotes castration-resistant prostate cancer. Nature. 2010 Mar;464(7286):302-5.

14.   Luo JL, Tan W, Ricono JM, Korchynskyi O, Zhang M, Gonias SL, Cheresh DA, Karin M. Nuclear cytokine-activated IKKα controls prostate cancer metastasis by repressing Maspin. Nature. 2007 Apr;446(7136):690-4.

15.   Woo, J.R. et al. (2014) Tumor infiltrating B-cells are increased in prostate cancer tissue. J. Transl. Med. 12, 30 47. Ou, Z. et al. (2015)

16.   Tumor microenvironment B cells increase bladder cancer metastasis via modulation of the IL-8/androgen receptor (AR)/MMPs signals. Oncotarget 6, 26065–26078

17.   Ou Z, Wang Y, Liu L, Li L, Yeh S, Qi L, Chang C. Tumor microenvironment B cells increase bladder cancer metastasis via modulation of the IL-8/androgen receptor (AR)/MMPs signals. Oncotarget. 2015 Sep 22;6(28):26065.

18.   Lund FE. Cytokine-producing B lymphocytes—key regulators of immunity. Current opinion in immunology. 2008 Jun 1;20(3):332-8.

19.   Balkwill F, Montfort A, Capasso M. B regulatory cells in cancer. Trends in immunology. 2013 Apr 1;34(4):169-73.

20.   Zhang Y, Gallastegui N, Rosenblatt JD. Regulatory B cells in anti-tumor immunity. International immunology. 2015 Oct 1;27(10):521-30.

21.   Bodogai, M. et al. (2015) Immunosuppressive and prometastatic functions of myeloid-derived suppressive cells rely upon education from tumor-associated B cells. Cancer Res. 75, 3456–3465

22.   Zhang, Y. et al. (2013) B lymphocyte inhibition of anti-tumor response depends on expansion of Treg but is independent of B-cell IL-10 secretion. Cancer Immunol. Immunother. 62, 87–99

23.   Tobon, G. J., Izquierdo, J. H. & Canas, C. A. B lymphocytes: development, tolerance, and their role in autoimmunity-focus on systemic lupus erythematosus. Autoimmune Dis. 2013, 827254 (2013).

24.   Xie M, Ma L, Xu T, Pan Y, Wang Q, Wei Y, Shu Y. Potential regulatory roles of microRNAs and long noncoding RNAs in anticancer therapies. Molecular Therapy-Nucleic Acids. 2018 Dec 7;13:233-43.

25.   Ahn H, Yang JM, Kim H, Chung JH, Ahn SH, Jeong WJ, Paik JH. Clinicopathologic implications of the miR-197/PD-L1 axis in oral squamous cell carcinoma. Oncotarget. 2017 Sep 12;8(39):66178.

26.   Biagi E, Rousseau R, Yvon E, Schwartz M, Dotti G, Foster A, Havlik-Cooper D, Grilley B, Gee A, Baker K, Carrum G. Responses to human CD40 ligand/human interleukin-2 autologous cell vaccine in patients with B-cell chronic lymphocytic leukemia. Clinical cancer research. 2005 Oct 1;11(19):6916-23.

27.   Wennhold K, Shimabukuro-Vornhagen A, von Bergwelt-Baildon M. B cell-based cancer immunotherapy. Transfusion Medicine and Hemotherapy. 2019;46 (1):36-46.

28.   Yuen GJ, Demissie E, Pillai S. B lymphocytes and cancer: a love–hate relationship. Trends in cancer. 2016 Dec 1;2(12):747-57.

Publisher: Eliva Press SRL

Email: info@elivapress.com

www.ingramcontent.com/pod-product-compliance
Lightning Source LLC
Chambersburg PA
CBHW070130240526
45468CB00002BA/826

Una ventana a la innovación

Jose Gregorio Silva
cheo@ula.ve

Primera versión: Diciembre de 2008

Primera edición impresa: Febrero 2010

Imágenes: Julia González

Portada y contraportada: Miguel Mora y María Dugarte

4

Agradecimiento de la Fundación Ideas

Una ventana a la Innovación ha sido ha sido un proyecto promovido con el objetivo de brindar, a cualquier persona que desee llevar adelante una iniciativa empresarial o social, la oportunidad de orientar la mirada hacia el extraordinario mundo de la innovación.

La Fundación Ideas ofrece este contenido como un módulo dentro de la "**Cátedra Virtual de Emprendimiento**", desde donde son accesibles los textos de este pequeño libro y muchos materiales complementarios adicionales en forma completamente gratuita. Invitamos a los interesados a visitarnos en **http://www.ideas.com.ve**.

Agradecemos en primer lugar a José Gregorio Silva, profesor de la Universidad de los Andes y Director de la Corporación Parque Tecnológico de Mérida (CPTM), quien desarrolló el contenido del módulo y el trabajo de búsqueda e identificación de fuentes complementarias de información para permitir al lector profundizar en los temas tratados. Sin su colaboración, dedicación y entusiasmo no hubiese sido posible incluir este módulo como parte de la Cátedra Virtual de Emprendimiento.

Igualmente, damos las gracias a *The Network Institute (TNI)*, por el aporte de las herramientas tecnológicas requeridas para montar el curso en línea y a *ERICSSON* y *EXITO-CATIVEN*, empresas que apoyaron y patrocinaron el desarrollo de la Cátedra Virtual de Emprendimiento.

Nuestra gratitud a todos

Fundación Ideas
http://www.ideas.com.ve

Agradecimientos del autor

El autor hace explícitos sus agradecimientos a sus compañeros de la Cátedra de Innovación, Organización y Asociatividad de la Corporación Parque Tecnológico de Mérida (CPTM) y la Universidad de Los Andes(ULA), Mérida, Venezuela: Genry Vargas, Marcos Rodríguez, Enrique Millán y Gilliam Aguirre.

Este agradecimiento se hace extensivo a múltiples instituciones que han organizado iniciativas conjuntas con esta cátedra, estimulando su desarrollo. Ellas son: Postgrado de Química en la Facultad de Ciencias y Postgrados de Computación y de Simulación de la Facultad de Ingeniería de la Universidad de Los Andes, Postgrado de Instrumentación de la Facultad de Ciencias de la Universidad Central de Venezuela, Postgrado en Gerencia de la Universidad de la Fuerza Armada, Centro de Excelencia en Ingeniería de Software (CEISoft). Por supuesto el agradecimiento del autor incluye a las personas que han venido participando en los talleres presenciales, con cuya experiencia se fraguó la presente iniciativa en línea, y a sus amigos y compañeros de equipo en las diversas aventuras emprendedoras impulsadas desde la ULA: Hacer-ULA, el Centro de Innovación Tecnológica de la ULA, RedUla y el Consejo de Computación Académica, HACER Sistemas, Escuela Latinoamericana de Redes, el Centro de Cálculo y Computación de Alto Rendimiento, CeCalcUla, CEISoft y la propia CPTM. Todas estas experiencias significaron importantes aprendizajes sobre innovación.

Agradecimientos muy especiales a la Fundación Ideas, por su confianza e interés, destacando con especial cariño a Laura Varela, quien coordinó la iniciativa de la publicación en línea. Y, desde luego, a mi familia, por su inspiración y apoyo.

Contenido

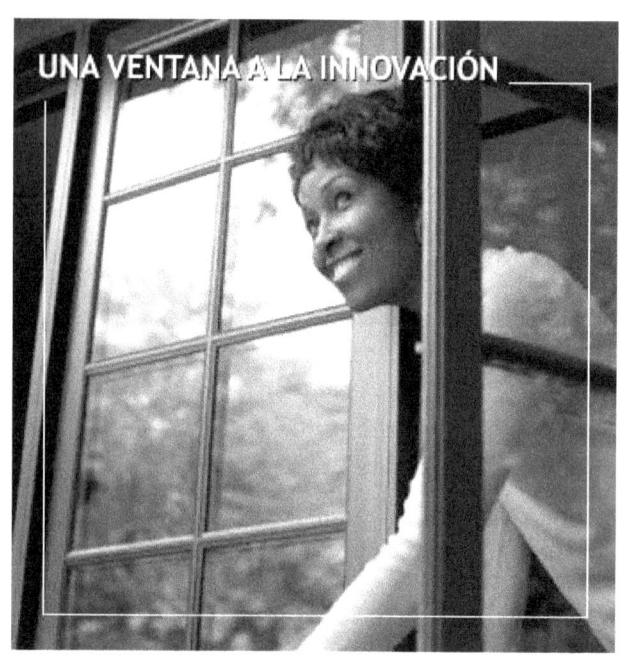

UNA VENTANA A LA INNOVACIÓN

Una ventana a la Innovación

El taller "Una ventana a la Innovación", con variantes significativas para adecuarlo a los distintos tipos de participantes, necesidades y organizaciones, lo hemos dictado numerosas veces en ambientes académicos y empresariales. Con la Fundacion Ideas (http://www.ideas.com.ve) hemos publicado una versión en línea. Nuestros lectores son bienvenidos a esta versión impresa. ¿Por qué usamos la metáfora de la ventana? ¿Qué podemos esperar de este taller?

La innovación es algo de lo que se habla bastante y en todos lados pero muchas veces con amplio desconocimiento sobre los conceptos involucrados. Se trata de uno de esos temas profundos e interesantes sobre los cuales con gran frecuencia, y lamentablemente, se habla muy superficialmente. Lo que pretendemos con este taller es ayudar a los que quieren iniciarse en el tema a tener una vista panorámica sobre el mismo, donde con comodidad nos apartamos de los lugares comunes y aprendemos a hacer una serie de distinciones importantes, esenciales en lo que respecta a innovación y que, a pesar de que son claves, muchas veces no se hacen y por eso se habla con impropiedad.

La innovación es también un tema fascinante y motivador. Una de esas áreas que cuanto más se conoce más se quiere conocer, y por eso es que con una buena introducción al mismo la motivación se dispara. Eso esperamos con este taller: que quienes trabajen con el material aprendan conceptos que definitivamente les ayudarán a distinguir no sólo lo que es innovación de lo que no lo es, algo que no es tan simple como parece, sino a manejar dimensiones más sofisticadas como las fuentes de la innovación y la relación con el conocimiento y con la organización. También el por qué son pocos los que tienen éxito con la innovación y cómo se gestiona el cambio de paradigmas.

La experiencia que tenemos con nuestros talleres presenciales es que los participantes disfrutan mientras aprenden y al final del taller expresan su agrado con la experiencia. Generalmente comentan que el conocimiento que adquirieron sobre innovación les sirve en muchos aspectos de su vida. Esperamos que esta versión impresa produzca el mismo tipo de satisfacciones y que al final nos descubramos manejando adecuadamente algunos conceptos interesantes y estemos definitivamente motivados a continuar aprendiendo sobre innovación.

La metáfora de la ventana: El conocimiento sobre innovación es demasiado amplio y escapa a lo que puede aprenderse leyendo un libro o toman do un taller, en línea o presencial. Lo que haremos en este caso es dibujar una ventana que nos dará una panorámica que esperamos sea tan interesante que estaremos tentados a mirar y volver a mirar a través de ella atraídos con esa magia que siempre tienen los ventanales que nos muestran un paisaje maravilloso.

Para cada persona y momento de lectura siempre hay tópicos que llaman más la atención que otros y por ello, para adaptarnos a públicos y contextos de lectura variados, desde la publicación en línea de este contenido, disponible en forma gratuita a través de http://www.ideas.com.ve, pueden consultarse enlaces que permiten obtener más información y caminos de profundización. Estos enlaces incluyen textos, paginas electrónicas y videos, seleccionados por el autor y asociados a cada capítulo del taller.

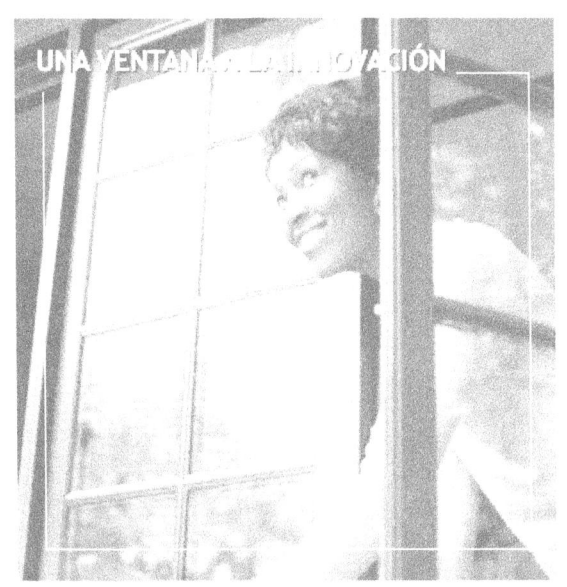

UNA VENTANA A LA INNOVACIÓN

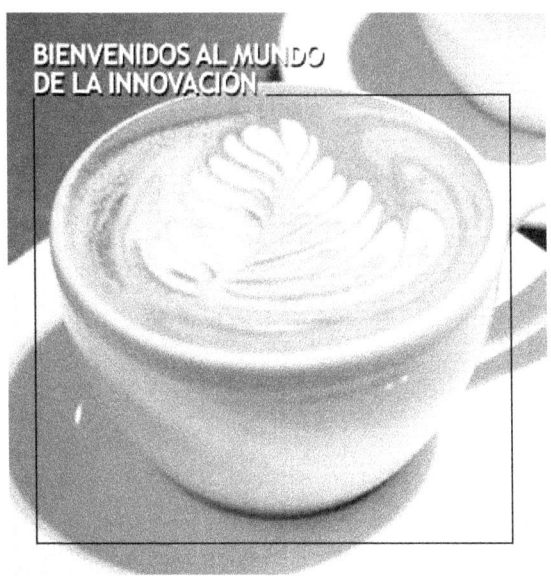

BIENVENIDOS AL MUNDO
DE LA INNOVACIÓN

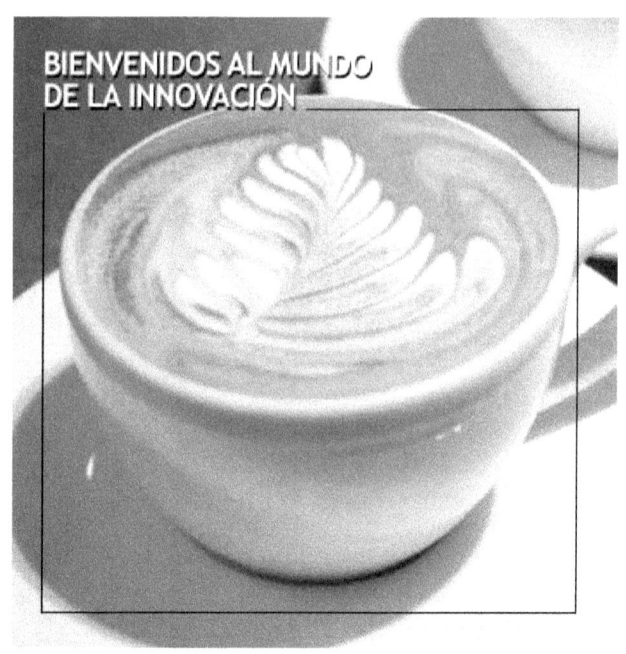

BIENVENIDOS AL MUNDO
DE LA INNOVACIÓN